The Coloring Review
of Neuroscience

The Coloring Review
of Neuroscience

Second Edition

D. Michael McKeough, Ed.D., P.T.
Associate Professor of Physical Therapy, Shenandoah
University; Physical Therapist, Winchester Medical
Center, Winchester, Virginia

Little, Brown and Company
Boston   New York   Toronto   London

To Regina, Emily, and Meghan
whom I love dearly

Library of Congress Cataloging-in-Publication Data

McKeough, D. Michael.
    The coloring review of neuroscience / D. Michael McKeough. — 2nd ed.
        p.   cm.
    Includes index.
    ISBN 0-316-56209-2
    1. Neurology—Programmed instruction.   2. Neurosciences—Programmed instruction.   Coloring books.   I. Title.
    [DNLM: 1. Nervous System—anatomy & histology—programmed instruction.   2. Nervous System—physiology—programmed instruction.   3. Nervous System—anatomy & histology—atlases.   WL 18.2 M478 1995]
    QP356.M38   1995
    612.8—dc20
    DNLM/DLC
    for Library of Congress   94-45666
                                                                                           CIP

Printed in the United States of America

HC

Editorial: Evan R. Schnittman, Rebecca Marnhout
Production Editor: Karen Feeney
Copyeditor: Libby Dabrowski
Proofreader: Gail Stewart
Indexer: Nancy Newman
Production Supervisor/Designer: Mike Burggren
Cover Designer: Linda Dana Willis and Patrick Newbery

Contents

Preface

In the years since the publication of the first edition of *The Coloring Review of Neuroscience* there have been dramatic new discoveries in the area of neurobiology. This new information, together with the desire to add a clinical component making the text more useful to the health-care professional, provided the incentive for this second edition.

The book is intended as a primer for the introductory neuroscience student. Because the first edition continues to be useful to many individuals, the same basic organization has been retained. Information is still presented by functional system rather than by anatomical region. Significant additions to the new edition include an introductory chapter that provides an overview of the nervous system from a functional perspective, a new chapter on the cranial nerves, updated information within each chapter, and an index. Many of the old illustrations have been retained, some of the busy ones have been simplified, and a few new ones have been added.

Any text is far from a solitary accomplishment. Among the many people who deserve thanks and recognition are the faculty, students, and staff in the Department of Physical Therapy at the Medical College of Georgia and the staff at Little, Brown and Company, including Evan Schnittman, Editor, Rebecca Marnhout, Development Editor, and Karen Feeney, Production Editor.

D.M.M.

Coloring Tips

1. Have a supply of 10 to 20 colors. Colored pencils are preferable to felt-tipped pens or wax crayons because they are easy to work with and will not leak through the page.

2. Read text material on the left-hand page before beginning to color, as this will provide an overview of the illustration and its parts.

3. Each illustration contains a list of terms indicating important structures. These structures and their functions have been discussed in the text. Color coding the term in the list and the structure in the illustration allows easy association of a structure with its proper name. Later, while studying, association of the structure with its name can be made by simply locating the same color in the illustration and in the bank of terms. The names of structures that cannot be colored in the illustration are printed in *italics*.

4. Each name in the list of terms is preceded by a letter and/or number. These letters/numbers are used to identify the corresponding structure in the illustration. The list of terms is printed in outline format. For example, in Chapter 1 the spinal cord is identified as "a" in the list of terms. Cervical, thoracic, lumbar, and sacral regions are subunits of the spinal cord and identified as "a1, a2, a3, and a4, respectively." If the larger unit cannot be color coded, its name is printed in *italics*.

5. At times all the structures to be colored in the illustration will not have an identifying label. This occurs in the case of symmetrical structures, where the unlabeled side is to be colored as well and where one or two labels imply that all similar structures should be colored. Some nonessential background or support structures are not labeled and need not be colored to understand how the system functions. However, if, when the illustration is complete, the uncolored structures seem conspicuous, feel free to color them.

6. It is the nature of anatomy that adjoining regions within a structure flow into each other, and individual regions are not always identified by distinct boundaries. At times this will create uncertainty as to where one color is to stop and another is to begin. Although there is no easy resolution to this problem, the text describes the function of individual structures and regions and may prove helpful in answering this type of question.

7. In some illustrations, texture or stippling has been used to highlight individual structures. The only significance of the texture is to help distinguish a particular structure from the surrounding anatomy.

8. If the same color is used for a particular structure each time it appears in an illustration, cross-referencing between illustrations will be made easier and a sense of continuity will be developed for that structure. Cross-referencing between illustrations is particularly effective when working with the internal structures of the brain, where the same structures appear repeatedly. This strategy will also help you to develop an appreciation for how individual structures change shape in different regions of the nervous system.

9. When beginning to color, use one color for each term and its associated structure. Coloring the terms first will help with cross-referencing and eliminate confusion that would stem from using the same color more than once in the same illustration.

10. Some illustrations contain solid lines, which represent regions or membranes. It may prove helpful to trace these lines with colors.

11. In general, use more neutral or lighter colors for larger structures and brighter or darker colors for smaller or more important structures.

The Coloring Review
of Neuroscience

1 Introduction and Overview

The human nervous system is the most complex structure known to exist on this planet. Neural science has experienced explosive growth in the last decade. The atmosphere in the field has become supercharged with the energy of anticipation as profound advances occur with increasing frequency. New technologies in imaging techniques have led to new understandings of neuronal structure and function. Insights into neurotransmitter substances have changed views of how information is transmitted. Advances in cell and molecular biology have led to new tests for neurological diseases while breakthroughs in transplantation and grafting techniques have led to new treatments. The field of neural science stands on the threshold of a new era. Much has changed recently and the potential for future growth is inspirational.

Overview

The function of the nervous system is to control behavior. For humans, the behavior that occupies the majority of waking hours is accomplishing goals. Goals are the desired outcome of the actions taken by the performer. Thus, the nervous system is controlling action that is produced intentionally because its consequences somehow help to produce a desired outcome. In accomplishing goals, the nervous system acts proactively by selecting a goal, monitoring sensory input to detect information essential to achieving the goal, and coordinating motor output to produce the desired outcome in the environment. That is to say, the nervous system is not passive. It does not spend time idly waiting to adapt to changes in the environment but rather interacts with and manipulates the environment in order to accomplish a preselected goal. The environment includes the external world around us and the internal world inside the body. Examples of goals that direct the activities of daily living include wishing to get out of bed, which requires some movement pattern to rise from the bed, or wishing to find a seat in which to eat lunch, which requires balancing a tray of food and drink while walking through a crowded cafe in search of an empty seat.

In striving to accomplish a goal, the nervous system performs three basic functions: sensation, perception,

and action. Sensory functions detect energy changes as they occur, perception involves interpreting the meaning of those changes, and purposeful action is produced by coordinated motor output. These three functions are performed by orchestrating the activity of an enormous number of individual cells called neurons. The human nervous system is estimated to contain approximately one billion neurons.

Neurons are specialized cells with the unique ability to generate and conduct electricity and they control behavior by acting collectively in functional systems. Networks of neurons are organized into functionally specialized systems dedicated to the control of specific aspects of behavior. In general, systems are either sensory, integrative, or motor based on the functions they regulate. A "system" is formed when a group of neurons coalesce to control a particular aspect of behavior. Systems generally consist of input, a control center, and output. Neurons can participate in more than one system at the same time.

Information Processing

For the nervous system, information is defined as a significant change in energy. Significant energy changes, such as the movement of objects and changes in temperature or light, occur almost constantly in the immediate environment both inside and outside the body. Specialized sensory receptors exist, each of which is most sensitive to changes in one specific form of energy. For example, the eyes are sensitive to changes in the frequency of light waves, the ears to changes in the frequency of sound waves, and the hair and skin to mechanical deformation. Sensory receptors inform the nervous system about changes as they are occurring.

Energy changes that occur inside the body are sensed by interoceptors located in the hollow viscera and perceived as cramps, pain, and fullness. Energy changes that occur outside the body are sensed by exteroceptors located near the body surface and perceived as touch, pressure, pain, temperature, odor, taste, sound, and light. Changes in body position are sensed by proprioceptors located within the inner ear, body wall, and extremities, and perceived as position, movement, vibration, and balance.

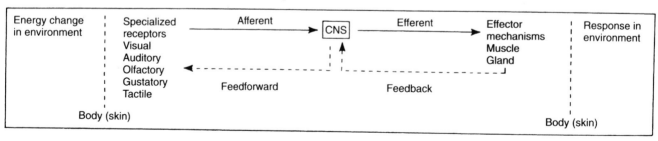

Fig. 1-1

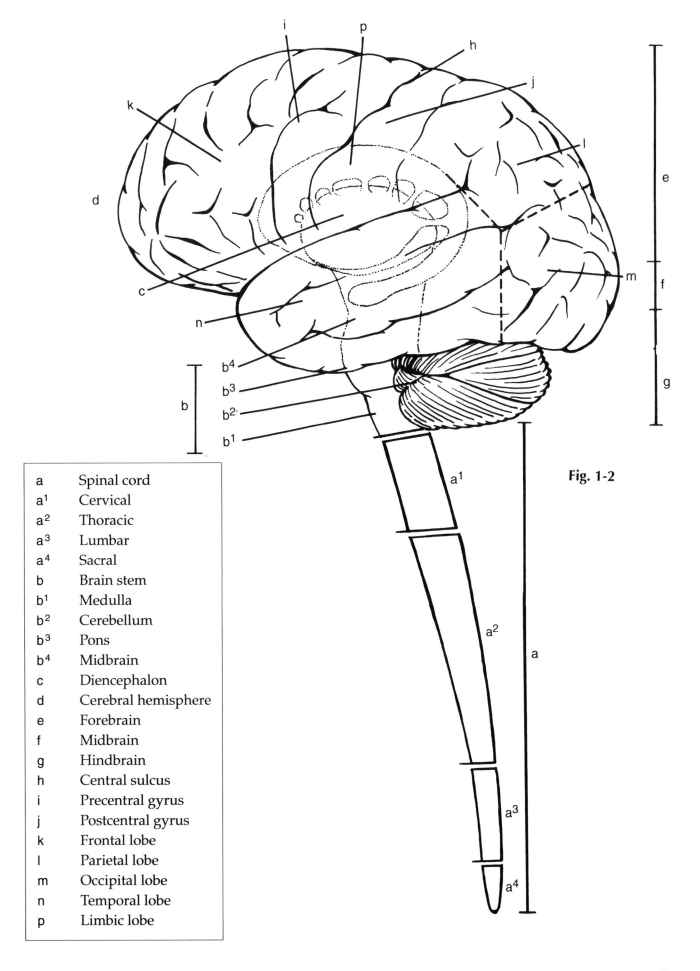

Fig. 1-2

a	Spinal cord
a^1	Cervical
a^2	Thoracic
a^3	Lumbar
a^4	Sacral
b	Brain stem
b^1	Medulla
b^2	Cerebellum
b^3	Pons
b^4	Midbrain
c	Diencephalon
d	Cerebral hemisphere
e	Forebrain
f	Midbrain
g	Hindbrain
h	Central sulcus
i	Precentral gyrus
j	Postcentral gyrus
k	Frontal lobe
l	Parietal lobe
m	Occipital lobe
n	Temporal lobe
p	Limbic lobe

3

The control of behavior is based on the ability of the nervous system to perform four basic information processing operations: (1) sense information from the environment, (2) transmit the information from the receptor to the central nervous system or from one location in the nervous system to another, (3) establish the meaning of that information (perception), and (4) select, plan, and initiate an appropriate response (Fig. 1-1). As the energy change is occurring, a specialized receptor senses it and relays the information to the central nervous system. Information transmitted toward the central nervous system is termed afferent. After analyzing and integrating sensory information, the central nervous system issues commands to the effector mechanisms (muscles or glands), which execute the desired response in the environment. Information transmitted away from the central nervous system is termed efferent.

The neurophysiological response process, from sensation to response initiation, is not a simple, unidirectional, linear process. Feedback and feedforward capabilities prevent the nervous system from being the passive recipient of stimulus change. Effector organs keep the central nervous system informed of their present condition through feedback mechanisms. Up-to-date knowledge of effector conditions is essential in order to accomplish a goal that requires movement. For example, if the goal is to pick up a pencil, the nervous system must know the position of the pencil in space and the position of the hand before it can determine how to move the arm. Smooth coordination of the reaching and grasping phases of the movement requires that the nervous system receive constant feedback about movement progress. The retrieval phase of the movement cannot begin before the pencil has been successfully grasped. The nervous system uses feedback from many systems (visual, tactile, and proprioceptive) to coordinate the different phases of the retrieval strategy. Every repetition of picking up a pencil is a novel solution to the motor problem of "getting the pencil." The nervous system does not have stored a predetermined movement pattern for achieving every goal but, instead, spontaneously creates an adaptive movement solution given the goal, strategy, and performance environment.

Similarly, sensory receptors are not the passive recipients of energy changes from the environment but act proactively, directed by the nervous system, in order to provide the information necessary to accomplish the goal. The orientation and sensitivity of sensory receptors are controlled through feedforward mechanisms. In the case of the eye, the nervous system actively aims the eyeball (globe) through voluntary contraction of extraocular muscles, focuses the image by adjusting the lens, and determines the level of illumination at the rods and cones by adjusting of the pupil.

Major Divisions of the Nervous System

Anatomically, the nervous system can be divided into two primary divisions: the central nervous system (CNS), which consists of the brain and spinal cord (Fig. 1-2), and the peripheral nervous system (PNS), which consists of the cranial nerves and spinal nerves. The central nervous system contains six main parts: the spinal cord, medulla, pons (and cerebellum), midbrain, diencephalon, and cerebral hemispheres. Table 1-1 lists the parts and the primary functions they control. The peripheral nervous system contains 31 pairs

Table 1-1 Functions of the Six Major Parts of the Nervous System

1. The spinal cord, the most caudal part of the CNS, is subdivided into four major segments. The spinal cord proper is responsible for receiving, analyzing, and transmitting information to and from the trunk and extremities. The individual segments are responsible for controlling restricted regions of the body: The cervical segment is responsible for the neck and arms, the thoracic segment is responsible for the trunk, the lumbar segment is responsible for the pelvis and legs, and the sacral region controls sphincter function.
2. The medulla oblongata lies directly above the spinal cord and contains the life-support centers responsible for controlling breathing, heart rate, and digestion.
3. The pons lies directly above the medulla and conveys information from the cerebral hemisphere to the cerebellum and from one cerebellar hemisphere to the other. The cerebellum lies behind the medulla and pons and below the brain. It is responsible for controlling the force and range of movement and is involved in learning motor skills.
4. The midbrain lies above the pons. It controls eye movement and coordinates visual and auditory reflexes. Together, the medulla, pons, and midbrain constitute the brain stem, which is responsible for controlling the sensory, motor, and special senses of the head via cranial nerves. Special senses include vision, audition, balance, and taste. Both ascending and descending projection pathways pass through the brain stem en route to their final destination. In addition, the brain stem also regulates levels of arousal and awareness. This is accomplished by a large group of diffusely organized nuclei referred to collectively as the reticular formation.
5. The diencephalon lies above the midbrain and consists of the thalamus and hypothalamus. The thalamus is a constellation of nuclei that relay most of the information reaching the cerebral cortex from the rest of the CNS. The hypothalamus regulates autonomic, endocrine, and visceral function.
6. The cerebral hemisphere lies above the diencephalon and consists of the cerebral cortex and subcortical structures: the basal ganglia, hippocampus, and amygdaloid nucleus. The basal ganglia help control movement, the hippocampus is involved in the process of memory storage, and the amygdaloid nucleus coordinates autonomic and endocrine responses with changes in emotional states.

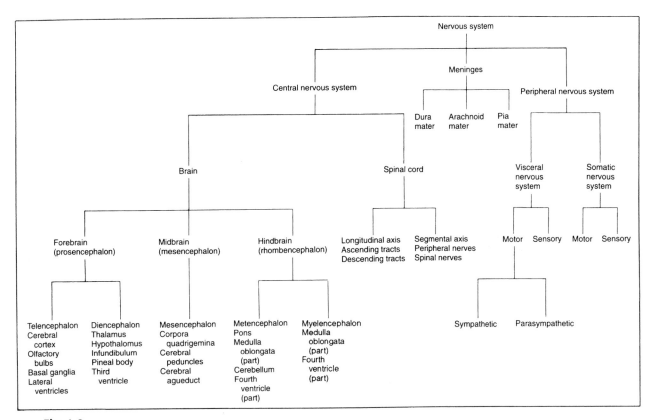

Fig. 1-3

of spinal nerves (8 cervical, 12 thoracic, 5 lumbar, 5 sacral, and 1 coccygeal) that pass through the vertebral column and serve the sensory and motor needs of the trunk and extremities, as well as 12 pairs of cranial nerves that pass through the skull and serve the sensory and motor needs of the head and neck. Figure 1-3 is a graphic diagram of all the components in the nervous system.

Functionally, the nervous system can also be divided into somatic and visceral components. The somatic nervous system is concerned with sensing and responding to changes in the external environment while the visceral nervous system senses and responds to changes in the environment inside the body (maintaining homeostasis). Visceral information remains largely at the subconscious level and the control of visceral response is mediated via automatic or subcortical reflexes. The visceral system contains sensory and motor divisions, both of which use a system of peripheral ganglia to regulate the function of effector organs. Visceral afferent fibers relay sensory information from the hollow organs of the body (stomach, bowel, bladder, vasculature, etc.). The visceral efferent system can be subdivided into sympathetic and parasympathetic divisions. Together, these two subdivisions comprise the autonomic system (that is, the autonomic system consists exclusively of visceral motor fibers). The sympathetic division controls the behaviors associated with arousal, such as those necessary to preserve life (fright, flight, fight, and procreation). The parasympathetic division controls restorative types of behavior, including eating, sleeping, and digestion.

The human nervous system, including all of its subdivisions, is organized along two major axes, a longitudinal rostral-to-caudal axis and a segmental dorsal-to-ventral axis (Fig. 1-4). During development, the longitudinal axis flexes almost 90 degrees, and several different terms are used to describe the orientation of structures in the mature human nervous system. In the brain, rostral means toward the nose, caudal toward the back of the head, dorsal toward the top of the head, and ventral toward the jaw. In the spinal cord, rostral means toward the head, caudal toward the tail, dorsal toward the back, and ventral toward the belly. Superior is used synonymously with dorsal and inferior synonymously with ventral.

Organizing Principles

Discussion of a few general organizing principles found repeatedly throughout the nervous system may assist in understanding the basic strategies that seem to control its functions.

Longitudinal and Segmental Systems

The nervous system is divided into right and left halves that, with a few important exceptions, are essentially symmetrical. Figure 1-5 shows the parts of the nervous system and the functions they control. The two halves of the brain (cerebral hemispheres) are connected to the body via longitudinal systems. The longitudinal systems are crossed such that the right hemisphere controls the somatic and visceral functions of the left side of the body (contralateral) and vice versa. Segmental systems (spinal and peripheral nerves as well as some cranial nerves) are uncrossed and control the somatic and visceral functions of restricted regions on the same side of the body (ipsilateral).

Each cerebral hemisphere is covered by superficial layers of cells known collectively as the cerebral cortex. Beneath the surface, each hemisphere contains projection fibers and nuclei (groups of cell bodies) with specialized functions. Each hemisphere is divided into five anatomically distinct lobes: frontal, parietal, occipital, temporal, and limbic (see Fig. 1-2). Originally, the frontal, parietal, occipital, and temporal lobes were named for the overlying bones of the skull. The limbic lobe is located deep within the hemisphere. Each lobe is responsible for controlling specialized functions. The frontal lobe controls movement, judgment, and personality; the parietal lobe controls sensory systems; the occipital lobe controls vision; the temporal lobe controls hearing and memory; and the limbic lobe controls drive, motivation, and affect. On gross examination the hemispheres appear to be symmetrical; however, closer inspection reveals unique structures that help each hemisphere to control different functions.

The spinal cord contains a longitudinal axis, consisting of ascending and descending tracts, and a horizontal axis, consisting of segmental levels and the spinal nerves they control. Ascending tracts transmit sensory information from the spinal cord to higher centers in the brain. Descending tracts carry information from higher brain centers to segmental levels. Segmental levels control the sensory and motor functions for restricted regions of the body (dermatomes, myotomes, sclerotomes) via spinal and peripheral nerves.

Topographic and Somatotopic Organization

Topographic organization has to do with the spatial location of structures within the nervous system. Anatomically, the structures with similar functions are located together or in the similar places at different levels. For example, at each level of the spinal cord the neurons that transmit information about pain from the body are located in the lateral aspect. Taken collectively, these thousands of fibers form the spinothalamic tract, which, by virtue of its anatomy, is specialized in carrying information that arose from pain receptors located throughout the body. Afferent fibers from the sacral region enter the tract first, followed by fibers from the lumbar, thoracic, and cervical regions. Within the tract, fibers originating in lower regions are pushed laterally by fibers entering from successively higher levels. Thus, the tract also has a somatotopic organization (see Fig. 11-2); that is, the body parts can be mapped on the tract. Similar topographic and somatotopic organization is found throughout the nervous system in sensory, motor, and visceral systems such

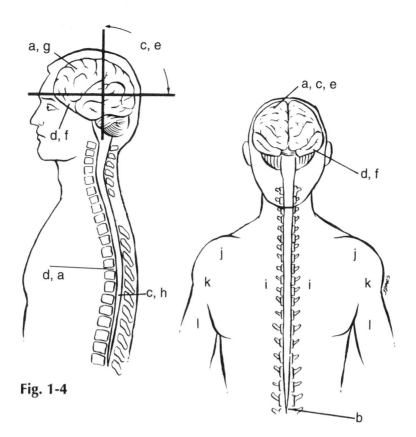

Fig. 1-4

a	Rostral
b	Caudal
c	Dorsal
d	Ventral
e	Superior
f	Inferior
g	Anterior
h	Posterior
i	Medial
j	Lateral
k	Proximal
l	Distal

that the spatial relationship of the body parts or peripheral receptor fields is maintained throughout the nervous system. However, not all body parts or receptive fields are represented with equal space. The areas with the greatest control or acuity are represented by a disproportionately large area because of the large number of neurons and synapses dedicated to their control. Probably the most famous example of topographic and somatotopic organization is the homunculus of the primary motor cortex (see Fig. 11-1.)

Phylogenetic Organization

During evolution of the nervous system, old structures were retained and new structures were added to the outside. With the addition of each new structure, a dramatically changed nervous system with new functions and new organizational relationships was created, what Konrad Lorenz called "fulguration." The result of these evolutionary changes is a phylogenetic organization where the oldest structures, those concerned with sustaining life, are located deep in the reticular core of the brain stem (sometimes referred to as the inner tube) and the newest structures (such as the cortex) and the fastest, most highly differentiated systems (dorsal column medial lemniscal system and lateral corticospinal tract) are located on the surface (sometimes referred to as the outer tube). The newest structures are the most sensitive to oxygen deprivation and the first to become injured due to ischemia.

Clinical Aspects

Pathological lesion of the nervous system produces systematic symptoms and signs that reflect the structure and function of the system within which the lesion is located. Irritative lesions such as inflammation will increase function within a given system, such as increased pain sensation, while destructive lesions will decrease function in that system, such as the inability to sense pain. For example, damage of the primary motor cortex in one cerebral hemisphere produces an inability to move the opposite side of the body. This symptom indicates that the motor cortex is involved in the control of movement and that the system for exerting that control is crossed. Complete transection of a spinal nerve produces the inability to move, sense, or control the visceral functions in a restricted region on the same side of the body. Interpretation of these symptoms indicates that spinal nerves are involved in the control of movement, sensation, and visceral function. The system for controlling these functions is uncrossed and it only controls a particular region on the same side of the body. Lesions and their effects are discussed here to provide additional, clinically relevant, information of how the nervous system is organized.

If a lesion occurs in one cerebral hemisphere, such as a cerebrovascular accident (CVA), the primary sensory and motor effects of the lesion will be seen in the opposite side of the body. Both motor and sensory symptoms and signs occur on the side opposite the lesion because the primary anatomical pathways connecting the brain and body (longitudinal systems) cross sides (Fig. 1-5). The specific symptoms and signs produced by a lesion will depend on which areas of the nervous system were affected.

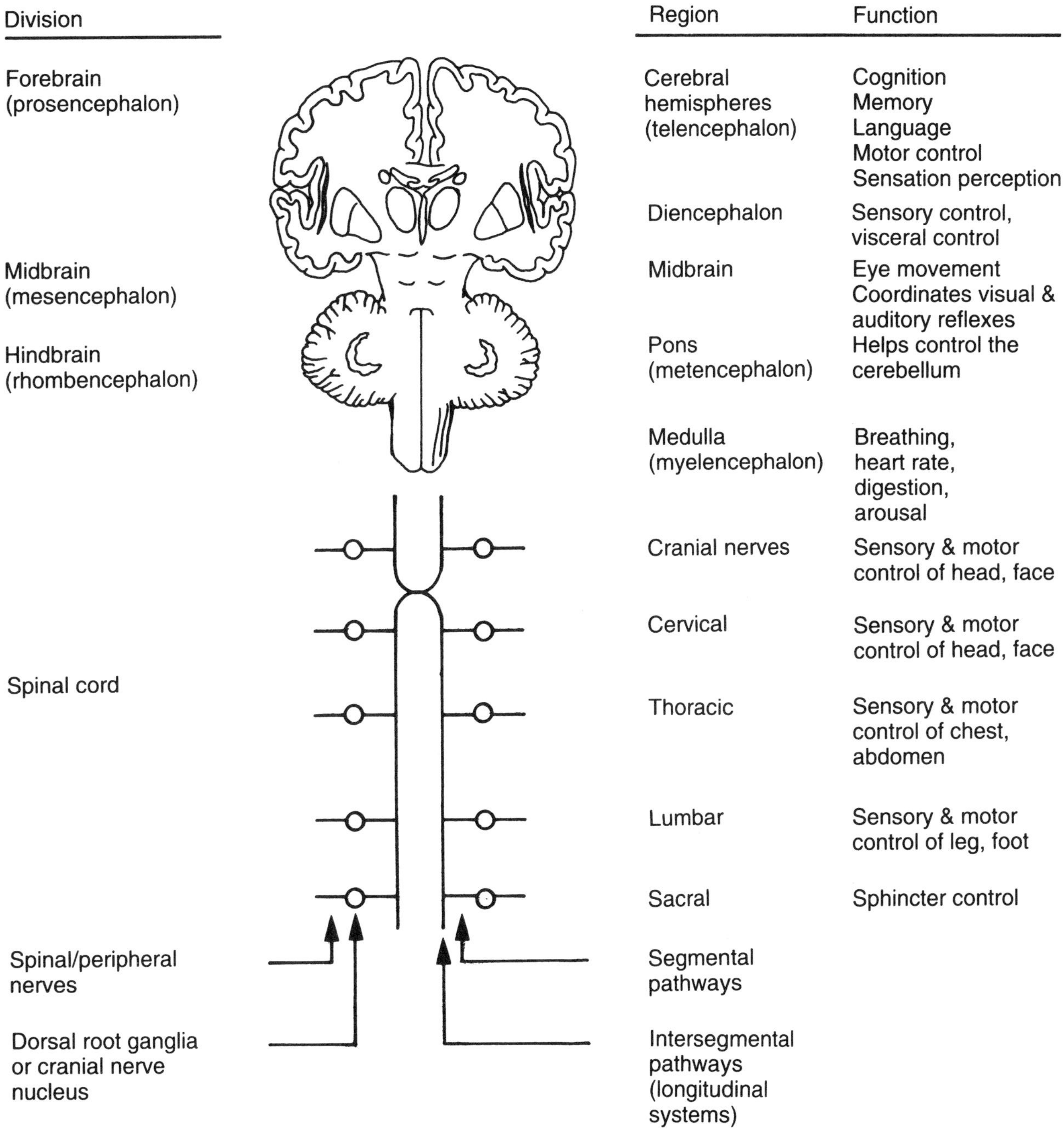

Division		Region	Function
Forebrain (prosencephalon)		Cerebral hemispheres (telencephalon)	Cognition Memory Language Motor control Sensation perception
		Diencephalon	Sensory control, visceral control
Midbrain (mesencephalon)		Midbrain	Eye movement Coordinates visual & auditory reflexes
Hindbrain (rhombencephalon)		Pons (metencephalon)	Helps control the cerebellum
		Medulla (myelencephalon)	Breathing, heart rate, digestion, arousal
		Cranial nerves	Sensory & motor control of head, face
		Cervical	Sensory & motor control of head, face
Spinal cord		Thoracic	Sensory & motor control of chest, abdomen
		Lumbar	Sensory & motor control of leg, foot
		Sacral	Sphincter control
Spinal/peripheral nerves		Segmental pathways	
Dorsal root ganglia or cranial nerve nucleus		Intersegmental pathways (longitudinal systems)	

Fig. 1-5 Schematic representation of the neuron system showing the four major divisions with the regions and the functions controlled by each.

2 The Neuron

Overview

Individual cells with the ability to generate and conduct electrical signals (neurons) are the basic unit from which the nervous system is constructed. Neurons are prototypes of the system at large and perform the same four information processing operations: reception, analysis, transmission, and response. Individual neurons are networked together into functional systems dedicated to the control of a particular aspect of behavior. Neurons communicate at specialized signaling junctions called synapses. Through the activity of neurons, the nervous system is able to command muscles to produce a desired change in the external environment. Damage to neurons is the mechanism underlying behavioral deficits following neurological injury, and recovery of the neuron is the mechanism that underlies functional return when it occurs.

Functions and Mechanisms

The function of the nervous system is to control behavior, and it does so by orchestrating the activity of an enormous number of individual cells called neurons (approximately one trillion, 10^{12}). Essentially, the nervous system is an electronic signaling system and the neuron is its smallest functional unit. The nervous system portrays information as transient electrical activity along a neuron. By organizing the activity of individual neurons into functional systems, the nervous system is able to monitor, interpret, and respond adaptively to events inside and outside the body. Each neuron is a miniature model of the nervous system and performs the same functions as the system at large: (1) reception and integration of information, (2) analysis of information, (3) transmission of information, and (4) initiation of a response or output. These four information processing functions are performed in morphologically distinct regions of the neuron (Fig. 2-1).

Information Processing and the Neuron

Information is received and integrated by the cell body and dendrites (receptive region). Integration occurs automatically as successive input interacts with the membrane potential at the time of arrival. Information is analyzed at the axon hillock, a specialized portion of the axon where an action potential is initiated if the critical threshold is reached (analytical region). Information is transmitted from one location in the nervous system to another as action potentials along the axon (transmissive region). A response is initiated at the presynaptic terminals (output region). Neurons are capable of producing a response in a target cell, either a postsynaptic neuron or an effector organ (muscle or gland).

The cell body (or soma) is the metabolic center of the neuron, responsible for synthesizing proteins that are then transported throughout the cell via axoplasmic flow (Fig. 2-2D). All parts of the cell depend on the products produced in the cell body and delivered via transport tubules. Transport is vital both away from (orthograde) and toward (retrograde) the cell body. Orthograde transport delivers materials that are only produced in the cell body but are required distally, while retrograde transport delivers to the cell body metabolites produced peripherally and trophic substance that has flowed backward across the synapse (retrograde direction).

Disruption of the transport systems is one of the mechanisms by which neurons are lesioned and the behavior supported by neuronal function is impaired. Specifically, the impaired function and widely dispersed lesions seen in patients with closed head injury are due to disruption of axonal transport. (See the clinical aspects section of this chapter for a more detailed discussion of this issue.)

The cell body usually gives rise to two types of cell processes, dendrites and axons (Fig. 2-2). Dendrites are delicate, cylindrical extensions of the cell body that greatly increase the surface area of the receptive segment of the cell. Along the receptive region, information in the form of transient electrical signals moves from the dendrites toward the cell body and from the cell body to the axon. The axons of multiple neurons are grouped together to form nerves and nerve tracts.

In addition to receiving incoming information, the receptive region is responsible for integrating this input. Integration of incoming information occurs continuously along the cell membrane as successive input changes the electrical potential of the membrane. Analysis of the integrated information is performed at the axon hillock by comparing the changing membrane potential with the critical electrical threshold. If, and only if, the changing membrane potential exceeds the critical threshold will an action potential be initiated at the axon hillock (all-or-none principle). Changing electrical potentials that fail to exceed threshold are short-lived. Homeostasis and a resting membrane potential are quickly restored and no action potential is initiated.

Once an action potential has been initiated, it is transported along the axon to its intended destination without loss of electrical power (nondecremental conduction). Thus, the axon forms the transmissive region of the neuron. Each cell body gives rise to only one axon, the diameter of which varies in proportion to cell size. Large-diameter axons are covered by nonneural,

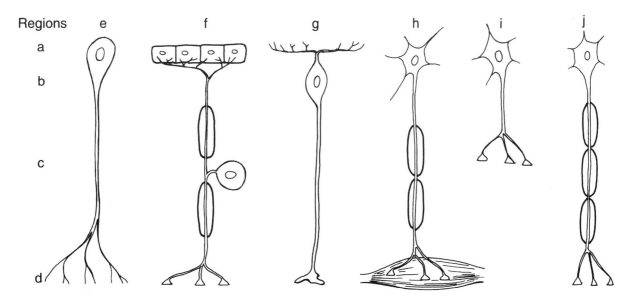

Fig. 2-1

a	Receptive region
b	Analytical region
c	Transmissive region
d	Output region
e	Unipolar neuron
f	Sensory neuron (pseudo-unipolar)
g	Bipolar neuron
h	Motor neuron
i	Local interneuron
j	Projection interneuron

electrically insulating myelin (Schwann or oligodendrocyte) cells (Fig. 2-2B,C). Schwann cells are found only in the peripheral nervous system, and oligodendrocytes are found only in the central nervous system. Myelin insulates because it is a lipid-based, nonconducting material. Myelination increases conduction velocity along the axon because the myelin sheath is interrupted intermittently at sites called nodes of Ranvier, and the action potential is transmitted along the axon by "jumping" from node to node (saltatory conduction, Fig. 2-2). Axonal transmission is fast because of saltatory conduction and nondecremental because the action potential is rejuvenated to its original strength at each successive node.

Near its end, the axon divides into multiple branches (telodendria) that form the output region of the neuron. The distal segment of each telodendria swells to accommodate the specialized structures housed in the presynaptic terminal, or terminal bouton (Fig. 2-2A). Most notable are the mitochondria and vesicles. Mitochondria produce the energy necessary to transport vesicles to the presynaptic terminals where they release neurotransmitter substance into the cleft separating presynaptic and postsynaptic cells. Neurotransmitter substance, the output product of neuronal activity, is taken up by receptor sites on the postsynaptic cell, where it produces a response. In neurons, neurotransmitter substance changes membrane permeability; in muscle, it produces a contraction; and in glands, it produces secretion.

Synaptic Communication

Communication between neurons usually occurs at specialized signaling junctions called synapses (Fig. 2-2A). The arrival of an action potential at the presynaptic terminal causes vesicles to migrate to specialized release sites (active zones), fuse with the surface membrane, burst, and release transmitter substance into the synaptic cleft. Neurotransmitter substance released into the cleft then migrates passively across the cleft, where it interacts with specialized receptor sites on the postsynaptic membrane. The arrival of transmitter substance at the receptor site changes the permeability and therefore the resting potential of the postsynaptic membrane. Through the transduction of energy from electrochemical on the presynaptic membrane to chemical in the cleft and back to electrochemical on the postsynaptic membrane, information is passed from one neuron to another. Given their physiology, synapses act as one-way gates determining that the flow of information within a functional system is unidirectional.

The molecular structure of the transmitter substance is one important factor determining which transmitter substance is taken up by which postsynaptic receptor site. Transmitter substance interacts with receptor sites in a key-and-lock type arrangement; that is, the spatial or structural configuration of the transmitter molecule must match the shape of the opening in the receptor site in order for the transmitter substance to be taken up. Any change in the configuration of the transmitter molecule or the receptor site will prevent uptake, and thus no postsynaptic reaction will occur.

Types of Synapses

The receptive region of each neuron is virtually covered with thousands of synaptic connections. Because most synapses originate from the axon of the presynaptic neuron, synapses are usually classified by their location on the postsynaptic cell. Most commonly, synapses are formed on the dendrite of the postsynaptic neuron (axodendritic). Less commonly, synapses occur on the soma (axosomatic) or axon (axoaxonic) of the postsynaptic neuron (Fig. 2-3).

Information Processing and Functional Systems

Because of their structure and function, synapses determine that the flow of information within the nervous system is unidirectional. Vesicles in the presynaptic neuron and receptor sites in the postsynaptic neuron form a one-way gate that regulates the flow of information from the presynaptic neuron to the postsynaptic neuron. Neurons are organized into functional systems in a serial configuration. For example, some of the most clinically relevant sensory systems consist of a three-neuron projection system (see Fig. 11-1). The first-order neuron projects from the sensory receptor in the periphery into the central nervous system, probably at the level of the spinal cord. Second-order neurons project from the spinal cord up to the brain, specifically, an important sensory integration station called the thalamus. Third-order neurons project from the thalamus to the cortex, which is the highest level of the central nervous system. This serial organization of neurons into a functional system is a fundamental organizing principle and/or information processing strategy that is used repeatedly throughout the nervous system.

In addition to serial processing of information within a given functional system, the nervous system shares or integrates information between systems through a strategy called parallel processing (Fig. 2-4). Because each neuron has many telodendria, its information can be shared with more than one postsynaptic neuron and, therefore, more than one functional system. When a neuron forms synaptic connections with many postsynaptic neurons, that is called divergence. When many neurons form postsynaptic connections with a single neuron, that is called convergence. Divergence can be used to disperse information from one system to many different systems and is common in sensory or input regions of the nervous system. Convergence can be used to integrate information from many different systems to a single system and is common in motor or output regions of the nervous system.

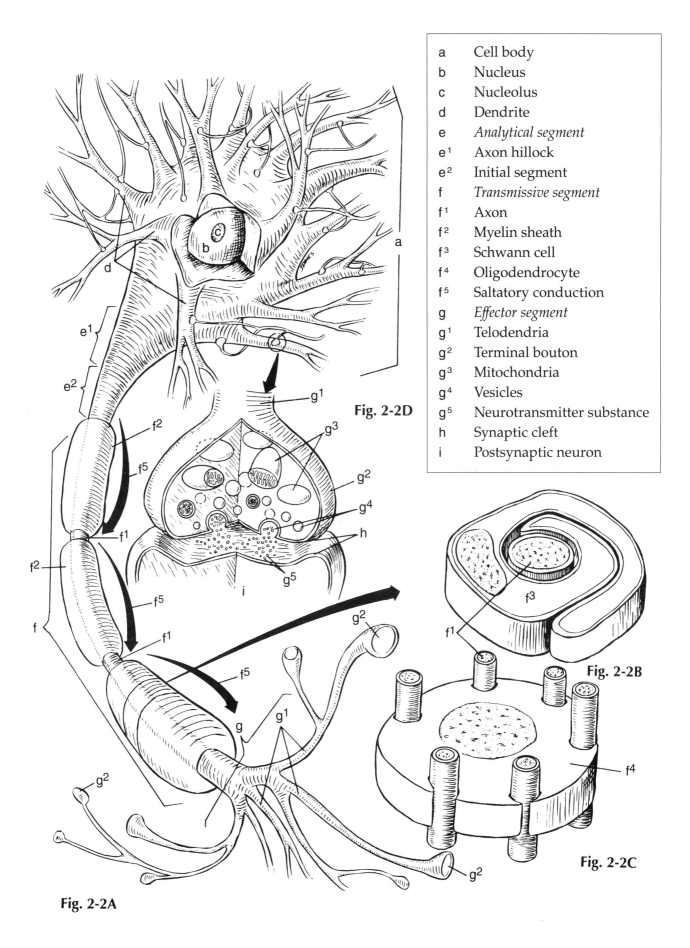

a	Cell body
b	Nucleus
c	Nucleolus
d	Dendrite
e	*Analytical segment*
e¹	Axon hillock
e²	Initial segment
f	*Transmissive segment*
f¹	Axon
f²	Myelin sheath
f³	Schwann cell
f⁴	Oligodendrocyte
f⁵	Saltatory conduction
g	*Effector segment*
g¹	Telodendria
g²	Terminal bouton
g³	Mitochondria
g⁴	Vesicles
g⁵	Neurotransmitter substance
h	Synaptic cleft
i	Postsynaptic neuron

Fig. 2-2D

Fig. 2-2B

Fig. 2-2C

Fig. 2-2A

Divergence and convergence are also fundamental organizing principles and/or information processing strategies that are used repeatedly throughout the nervous system.

Types of Neurons

The feature that most dramatically distinguishes one neuron from another is shape, specifically the number and form of its processes. Structurally, neurons are classified into three major groups on the basis of the number of processes (poles) emanating from the cell body: unipolar, bipolar, and multipolar (see Fig. 2-1). Unipolar neurons have a round cell body that gives rise to one primary process that may split into many branches. One branch forms the axon and the other branches form the dendritic or receptive segment of the cell. No dendrites emerge from the cell body of these neurons. Unipolar cells predominate in the nervous system of invertebrates but also occur in certain ganglia of the vertebrate autonomic nervous system.

Bipolar neurons have a round cell body that gives rise to two processes: The distal process or dendrite conveys information toward the cell body, and the proximal process or axon conveys information from the cell body toward the central nervous system. Most bipolar neurons are found in sensory systems including the visual and olfactory systems. The first-order neurons in the somatic sensory system, those that convey information about touch, pressure, and pain, form a special class of bipolar cells. The distal axon extends to the periphery, where it innervates a sensory receptor, and the proximal axon extends into the spinal cord.

Multipolar neurons comprise the largest class of cells in the vertebrate nervous system. These cells have two or more dendrites and a single axon that emerge from the cell body. The size and shape of multipolar cells vary enormously from a spinal motor neuron to a cerebellar Purkinje cell. The number of dendrites and the extent of dendritic branching are proportional to the number of synaptic connections received by that cell. A typical spinal motor neuron receives approximately 10,000 synaptic connections, 20 percent of which occur on the cell body and 80 percent of which occur on dendrites. The Purkinje cell of the cerebellum, which has the most richly branching dendritic system of any neuron, receives as many as 150,000 synaptic connections, which makes it superbly designed to integrate information.

Functionally, neurons can be classified into three major groups: sensory, motor, and interneuronal (see Fig. 2-1). Sensory neurons are also called afferent because they convey sensory information from the periphery into the central nervous system. The information transmitted along sensory neurons is used to formulate conscious perception and forms the basis for coordinating voluntary movement. Motor neurons are also called efferent because they convey commands away from the central nervous system to effector organs (muscles and glands). Interneurons constitute by far the largest class of neurons in the nervous system and include all the remaining cells that are not specifically sensory or motor. Interneurons have two primary functions and come in two primary cell types. The first function is to process information locally and is performed by neurons with rich dendritic trees and short axons (local interneurons). The second function is to transmit information between distant sites within the central nervous system and is performed by neurons with long axons. The axons of transmission neurons form tracts, fiber bundles, and projection systems in the spinal cord and brain (projection interneurons).

Functional Systems

Functional systems consist of specialized sensory receptors, dedicated projection pathways, control centers, and efferent neurons, all devoted to the control of a particular function. Functional systems are determined not by the unique characteristics of neurons within that system, but by the specific interconnections between relatively stereotyped nerve cells. For example, tactile discrimination and pain are processed by completely separate functional systems, though both systems originate from sensory receptors in the periphery, and project through the spinal cord to the same nucleus in the thalamus and onto the same region in the cortex. The unique interconnections between similar types of neurons are what make the two systems functionally distinct. The same is true for the special senses and movement. The specific pattern of interconnections, not the unique characteristics of the neurons, permits a neural network to develop its functional capability.

Clinical Aspects

Clinical problems with neurons arise from ischemic, traumatic, toxic, and degenerative sources as well as from abnormal growth. The reaction of neurons to damage varies dramatically. Damage that destroys the cell body or axon hillock of a neuron leads invariably to the death of the cell. A neuron may survive damage to its axon if it is able to restore functional connections with target cells. If its connections are not restored, the neuron will atrophy and die. When neurons in the adult nervous system die, they are not replaced. Neuronal death results in long-lasting or permanent loss of function. In the peripheral nervous system, damage is frequently reversible. Neurons are often able to regenerate axons and reestablish functional connections with target cells and thereby regain lost function. In the central nervous system, damaged axons do not reestablish functional connections with target cells; thus, there is no recovery of function following complete transection of the spinal cord. Any recovery of function following cerebrovascular accident is based on collateral sprouting from intact neurons and/or intact functional systems substituting for the lost function.

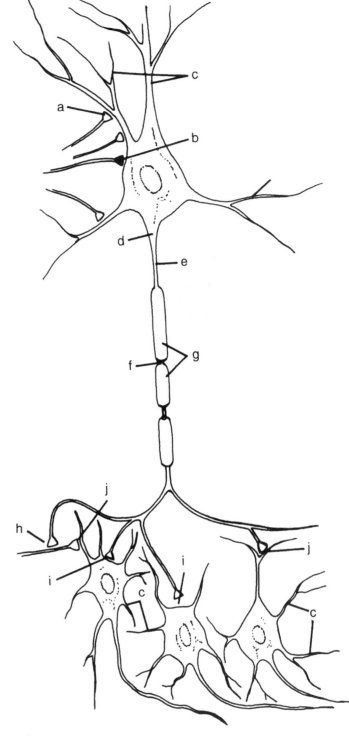

Fig. 2-3

a	Facilitatory terminal
b	Inhibitory terminal
c	Dendrites
d	Axon hillock
e	Axon
f	Node of Ranvier
g	Myelin sheath
h	Axoaxonic synapse
i	Axosomatic synapse
j	Axodendritic synapse

Injury to an axon is classified into three categories according to the extent of damage. The first is neuropraxia, of which there are two types. Transient neuropraxia is due to an ischemic block of conductivity and presents as a rapidly reversible loss of the function subserved by the nerve. An example of transient neuropraxia is the heavy, numb, tingling sensation in an extremity that has been maintained in a position such that the blood supply to the nerve has been interrupted. Delayed, reversible neuropraxia is due to demyelination and presents as a loss of function that recovers after a few weeks following remyelination. The second class of axonal injury, axonotmesis, is a complete interruption of the axon with loss of all functions subserved by that cell. Regeneration and recovery of function may occur following this type of injury (see discussion below). The third class, neurotmesis, is a complete interruption of the entire nerve fiber including myelin and connective tissue surrounding the nerve fiber (endoneurium; see discussion below).

Lesion of an axon (axonotmesis or axotomy) divides the neuron into proximal and distal segments (Fig. 2-5). Immediate and long-term changes occur in both segments. Immediately after injury, axoplasm leaks from the cut ends of both segments and synaptic transmission soon ceases. Shortly thereafter, the cut ends seal, swell, and retract from each other. Glial cells, including fibrous astrocytes, proliferate and form a glial scar around the damaged area. Within days, axonal degeneration progresses both away from (orthograde) and toward (retrograde) the cell body. Nonreversible, orthograde degenerative changes occur in the distal segment (wallerian degeneration) because the segment has been separated from the life-support systems provided by the cell body. Debris from the degeneration is removed by the phagocytic activity of macrophages in the peripheral nervous system and microglial cells in the central nervous system. In the peripheral nervous system, once the debris has been removed, Schwann cells occupy the space within the endoneurial sheath. The tubular process formed by the endoneurium functions as "a road map" to guide regenerating axonal sprouts, thereby greatly increasing the probability of reaching and reinnervating a target cell.

Degenerative changes also occur in the proximal segment (retrograde degeneration) but these changes are extremely variable. Retrograde degeneration usually involves the axon and its sheath for a distance of one or two nodes of Ranvier but may also involve the cell body. Depending on the extent of involvement of the cell body, retrograde degeneration may be reversible or it may lead to cell death. If the cell survives, the cell body undergoes characteristic morphological changes (chromatolysis) that include swelling of the cell body, peripheral displacement of the nucleus, and dispersion of the Nissl substance. Nissl substance or Nissl bodies are composed of portions of endoplasmic reticulum that produce the proteins and enzymes needed for neurotransmitters and cellular regeneration. Chromatolysis seems to be related to the formation of new protein for the purpose of repairing the cell and its damaged axon.

If the cell body and axon survive the damage, the proximal segment of the nerve fiber may begin the process of regeneration. Regeneration may begin as early as three hours after injury, at which time the tip of the proximal segment begins forming an enlarged growth cone. Between 10 and 40 axonal sprouts project from the growth cone and grow by pursuing the nerve growth factor secreted by the axonal sprout. If an axonal sprout enters the endoneurium, reinnervation and recovery of function usually follow if the target cell is not too far distant. The fact that each regenerating axon produces many new sprouts increases the chances of reinnervation. Should reinnervation occur, the successful sprout continues to develop and all other sprouts die. Remyelinization of a sprout begins only after successful reinnervation of a target cell and continues for 6 to 12 months.

Both sensory and motor neurons are only capable of reinnervating appropriate effector mechanisms (sensory neurons to sensory receptors and motor neurons to muscles and glands). However, the first alpha lower motor neuron (large-diameter motor neuron innervating skeletal muscle) to reach a muscle will reinnervate it, whether or not it is the appropriate type of motor neuron. This "winner takes all" strategy sometimes leads to complications during recovery. For example, if the flexor carpi ulnaris muscle (a flexor of the hand at the wrist) is reinnervated by a branch of the radial nerve (which only innervates extensors of the hand at the wrist), activity in the radial nerve will elicit extension of the hand at the wrist from the "normal" extensors and flexion of the hand at the wrist from the aberrantly reinnervated flexor muscle. No treatment or reeducation programs are effective under such circumstances. An equally severe but more common problem is seen in the post–nerve lesion dysesthesia, where aberrant sensory reinnervation results in a gentle touch of the skin being interpreted as persistently painful.

Recovery of function following nerve injury is painfully slow. Regeneration progresses at between 1 and 2 mm a day; reinnervation and remyelinization may take as long as 12 to 18 months. During this time the target tissue must be maintained in a viable state if functional return is to remain possible. A muscle that has atrophied or become contracted, or a joint that has become ankylosed, produces additional difficulties to the recovery of function. While waiting for reinnervation to occur, therapeutic treatment activities are directed at maintaining the integrity of target tissue. Electrical stimulation of denervated muscle is intended to maintain muscle integrity. Passive range of motion is intended to maintain joint integrity. Patient education, adaptation of activities of daily living, positioning, and splinting are used to prevent contractures and protect desensate structures. Electrodiagnostic testing, in the forms of nerve conduction velocity and electromyography, is used clinically to quantify the effects

Divergence   Convergence

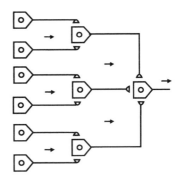

Fig. 2-4

of peripheral nerve lesion and regeneration. Once re-innervation has begun, therapeutic treatment activities are directed at maximizing recovery of function.

Transneuronal Lesion Effects

Axotomy also produces secondary effects. These effects seem to be based on interruption of the flow of trophic substances between the injured neuron and those making synaptic connections with it. Transneuronal or transsynaptic effects occur in both orthograde and retrograde directions (Fig. 2-5). Soon after axotomy, invading glial cells push the axon terminal away from the postsynaptic cell (orthograde direction), producing atrophy and denervation supersensitivity of that cell. Muscular atrophy and spasticity are examples of the secondary effects of axotomy following lesion of a lower motor neuron. Degenerative changes also occur in presynaptic neurons (retrograde direction) and have been shown to be due to the interruption of the axoplasmic transport of trophic substance backward across the synapse.

Aberrant Cell Growth

Neurotmesis, lesion of the entire nerve fiber including endoneural covering, is a very serious injury that requires surgical reattachment of the cut nerve ends if functional recovery is to occur. A frequent complication with neurotmesis is a neuroma or collection of aberrant axonal sprouts. Neuromas can be very painful because they may contain many pain fibers. They sometimes occur after limb amputation because the distal segment of the nerve is removed.

Tumors of aberrant cell growth is another clinical problem with the neuron. Because mature neurons have withdrawn from the mitotic cycle and no longer multiply, tumors of the nervous system (neoplasms) arise from nonneural tissue. Proliferation of glial or endoneural cells is a common source of neoplasms. In very rare circumstances, immature neurons produce tumors called neuroblastomas.

Demyelinating Lesions

A demyelinating lesion of the neuron is seen in multiple sclerosis (MS). The disease is caused by a lesion of the myelin sheath surrounding the axon that disrupts impulse propagation with a loss of the functions controlled by that cell. Lesions occur randomly throughout the central nervous system and the resulting symptoms and signs depend on the system affected. Magnetic resonance imaging (MRI) is used to diagnose the disease by revealing the scars produced by the lesions (plaques). No effective treatment for the disease currently exists; however, new medications have produced much better relief of some of the symptoms.

Neuronal Lesions in Closed Head Injury

Closed head injuries are produced by the application of powerful acceleration and deceleration forces to the head. As a result, the central nervous system experiences shear forces that stretch the nonelastic connective tissue surrounding the neuron (endoneurium). As the tissue stretches, it narrows the space available on the inside of the axon, which restricts or interrupts axoplasmic flow. In so doing, the stretching produces an axonotmesis with an accompanying loss of function. Because the shear force is experienced throughout the central nervous system, the resulting lesions are also widely distributed in many functional systems. The symptoms and signs of closed head injury characteristically include the involvement of multiple functional systems (motor, sensory, psychological, balance) from diverse locations and different segmental levels of the central nervous system.

Synaptic Blocks

Finally, many human diseases and some of the most deadly poisons function by disrupting chemical transmission between neurons and their target cells. Both postsynaptic and presynaptic blocks exist. Myasthenia gravis is an autoimmune disease in which antibodies are produced against acetylcholine (ACh) receptors in muscle. The muscular weakness that results can be reversed by drugs that inhibit acetylcholinesterase, the enzyme that degrades ACh. Curare produces its muscle-paralyzing effects with a similar ACh uptake blocking mechanism. The most poisonous snakes and electric eels inject neurotoxins that bind irreversibly to ACh receptor sites blocking any further uptake. Botulism, a potentially lethal form of food poisoning, produces its effects by a presynaptic block of ACh release as its mechanism of effectiveness.

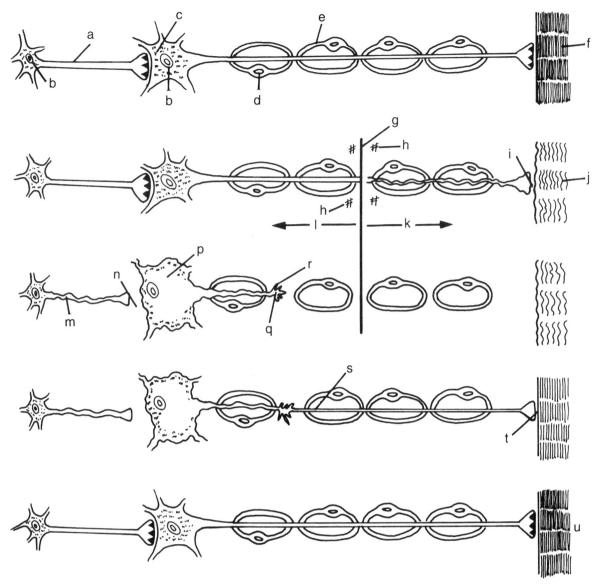

Fig. 2-5

a	Presynaptic neuron	l	Retrograde degeneration
b	Nucleus	m	Transneuronal degeneration
c	Nissl substance	n	Synaptic retraction
d	Schwann cell nucleus	p	Chromatolysis
e	Myelin	q	Growth cone
f	Muscle fiber	r	Axonal sprouts
g	Lesion	s	Axonal growth
h	Macrophage	t	Reinnervation
i	Terminal degeneration	u	Recovery of function
j	Muscle atrophy		
k	Wallerian (orthograde) degeneration		

3 Excitation, Conduction, and Transmission

Overview

In a resting state, the cell membrane maintains a dynamic disequilibrium between the chemical environments inside and outside the neuron, a condition referred to as the resting membrane potential. This disequilibrium exists between the concentrations of a few important chemicals in extracellular and intracellular fluid. Disruption of the resting membrane potential provides the basis for generating, conducting, and transmitting nerve impulses. When a nerve impulse travels the length of an axon and reaches the terminal bouton, it causes a neurotransmitter substance to be released from the presynaptic membrane. The transmitter substance diffuses passively across the synaptic cleft, where it interacts with and disrupts the resting membrane potential of the postsynaptic membrane. The amount of disruption will determine whether threshold will be reached in the postsynaptic cell. For threshold to be reached, individual synaptic events must be summed. Intervention into the process of synaptic transmission is the means by which some diseases, some medicines, and some of the most potent poisons achieve their effects.

Resting Membrane Potential

A nerve cell membrane actively maintains a separation between extracellular and intracellular fluids, which differ drastically in ionic concentrations. The extracellular fluid has much higher concentrations of sodium (Na^+) and chloride (Cl^-) than the intracellular fluid, and the intracellular fluid has much higher concentrations of potassium (K^+) and anions (Fig. 3-1). All ions contain an electrical charge; those with a positive charge are termed cations and those with a negative charge are anions. The difference in ionic concentrations between extracellular and intracellular fluid creates a concentration gradient, which is an energy source that allows ions to move from an area of higher concentration to one of lower concentration. The cell membrane is selectively permeable and allows potassium to diffuse more readily than the other ions. As potassium exits, leaving behind the nondiffusible anions, it creates a separation of positive and negative charges. The separation produces a voltage gradient, an energy source that, because of the attraction of oppositely charged ions, draws extracellular cations to the inside of the membrane and intracellular anions to the outside. The concentration and voltage gradients reach a dynamic equilibrium when the interior of the membrane is approximately 70 mV negative as compared to the exterior of the membrane (resting membrane potential). As long as the resting membrane potential is maintained, the concentration and voltage gradients provide an energy source for the movement of extracellular and intracellular ions and, thus, the conduction of a nerve impulse.

The cell membrane contains channels through which ions can move. Channels are macro protein molecules capable of changing their configuration in response to different signals (Fig. 3-1). Configurational change acts like opening and closing a gate. The channels located on the receptive segment of the cell open and close their gates in response to chemical signals. The channels located on the transmissive segment of the cell open and close their gates in response to changes in voltage. Some channels located throughout the cell are nongated, which permits both sodium and potassium ions to constantly "leak" through the cell membrane along their concentration and voltage gradients (sodium moves in and potassium moves out). "Leakage" is reversed by an active pumping process that operates continuously to return the two chemicals to their starting positions and thereby maintains the resting membrane potential. The pump exchanges sodium ions that have entered the cell for potassium ions that have escaped. This is accomplished by an intrinsic membrane protein, termed the sodium-potassium pump (Fig. 3-1). Each sodium-potassium pump harnesses the energy stored in adenosine triphosphate (ATP) to exchange three sodium ions on the inside of the cell for two potassium ions on the outside. Although pump density and operating rate vary with cell location and physiological demand, a typical small neuron contains perhaps a million sodium-potassium pumps with a capacity to move approximately 200 million sodium ions per second. This functional capacity is quite adequate to allow the pumps to keep the cell membrane "charged up" so that the cell can respond continuously.

Thus, the resting membrane potential or dynamic equilibrium that the cell membrane is constantly trying to achieve and maintain depends on three factors: selective permeability, which creates a disequilibrium between the concentrations of ions in the extracellular and intracellular fluid; concentration and voltage gradients, which provide the power to move ions during active states; and sodium-potassium pumps, which work to actively maintain or reestablish resting membrane potential. The primary factor affecting membrane potential is permeability. The arrival of neurotransmitter substance changes membrane permeability drastically by opening chemically gated channels, which permits ions to move freely along their concentration and voltage gradients.

Voltage-Gated Transmission

The transmissive segment of the cell contains voltage-gated channels. Channel gates open and close in

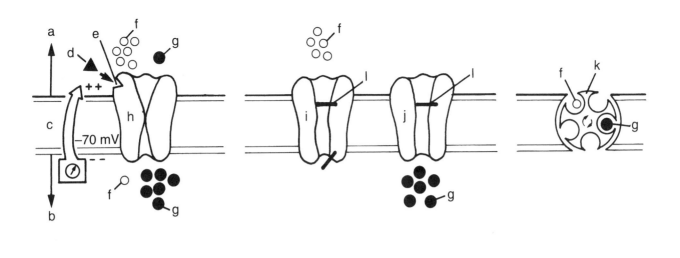

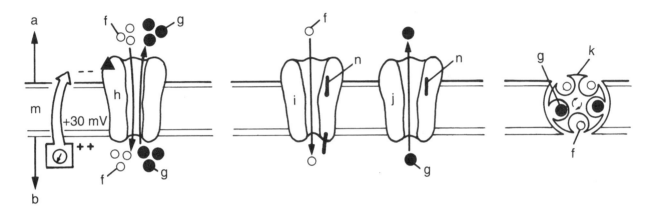

Fig. 3-1

a	Extracellular space
b	Intracellular space
c	Membrane in resting state
d	Neurotransmitter
e	Receptor site
f	Sodium
g	Potassium
h	Chemically gated channel
i	Voltage-gated sodium channel
j	Voltage-gated potassium channel
k	Sodium-potassium pump
l	Gate closed
m	Depolarized membrane
n	Gate open

response to voltage changes across the cell membrane (Fig. 3-1). When threshold is reached at the initial transmissive segment, voltage gates open, producing a drastic (all-or-none) change in membrane permeability. Open channels permit enough sodium to flood into the cell so that the polarity of the membrane reverses and the interior becomes positive with respect to the exterior. Inrushing sodium creates a flow of electrical current that penetrates the membrane in a local region and traverses longitudinally along the membrane. The effects of the longitudinal flow are strong enough to cause the opening of voltage-gated sodium channels in adjacent segments of the membrane. Sodium channels remain open just long enough for sodium to reach equilibrium, which occurs at about +30 mV. Because the movement of sodium ions is powered by the concentration gradient, which is zero when sodium has reached equilibrium, the nerve impulse will reach +30 mV at each node along the axon, thereby producing nondecremental conduction. When sodium channels close, potassium channels open, which allows potassium to rush out of the cell. The escaping potassium ions help to return the cell membrane to its resting state of −70 mV. The sharp positive and then negative change in the membrane potential is termed a spike or action potential, which is the electrical recording of a nerve impulse (Fig. 3-2).

The transmissive segment of the cell conducts each nerve impulse at the same amplitude, and, therefore, a frequency code is used to represent the information being carried along the axon. Frequency coding consists of neurons generating a train of impulses with a frequency that reflects the intensity of the stimulus. As stimulus intensity increases, discharge frequency increases, and vice versa.

Directly Gated Chemical Transmission

The receptive segment of the neuron contains chemically gated channels. When a particular molecule (a neurotransmitter substance) binds to the receptor site on the surface of the channel, the gates open (see Fig. 3-1). The neurotransmitter substance and receptor site on the channel interact in a key-and-lock type arrangement to open the channel gates and thereby change the permeability of the receptive segment of the neuron. The receptor, not the transmitter, determines whether the postsynaptic response is excitatory or inhibitory. An excitatory response depolarizes the postsynaptic membrane (excitatory postsynaptic potential, or EPSP). This is achieved when channels open and allow positively charged ions to flow into the cell and decrease the resting membrane potential (−70 mV to −50 mV). An inhibitory response hyperpolarizes the postsynaptic membrane (inhibitory postsynaptic response, or IPSP). This is achieved when channels open and allow negatively charged chloride ions to flow into the cell and increase the resting membrane potential (−70 mV to −90 mV).

The amplitude of the postsynaptic potential is proportional to the amount of neurotransmitter released (graded response), and it diminishes with the distance traveled from the receptor site (decremental conduction). The graded, local, and decremental properties of the postsynaptic potential differ from the transmission properties of the action potential, which are all-or-none, self-propagating, and nondecremental. Table 3-1 compares the transmission properties of the receptive and transmissive segments of the cell.

The postsynaptic effect of neurotransmitter substance is limited in both amplitude and duration. The amount of transmitter substance released as the result of a single presynaptic nerve impulse is incapable of depolarizing the postsynaptic membrane enough to reach critical threshold. Thus, if threshold is to be reached and the impulse passed along by the postsynaptic neuron, summation of postsynaptic effects is necessary. Two types of summation exist: temporal and spatial. Temporal summation occurs in the postsynaptic membrane as the result of the number of impulses and the time between impulses occurring at a single synapse (Fig. 3-3). The postsynaptic effects of a given neurotransmitter substance are constant and additive, meaning that equal quantities of transmitter substance always have the same effect and these effects may be summed. If 10,000 molecules of transmitter substance (the amount released by a single nerve impulse) depolarize the postsynaptic membrane 10 mV, they will do so every time they arrive, whether the membrane is in a resting state or immediately subthreshold. The arrival of each nerve impulse drives the postsynaptic membrane 10 mV closer to threshold, presuming that the response was an EPSP. Postsynaptic effects are short-lived because enzymes that are stored in the receptor sites decompose the transmitter substance. This helps to close the channels, and the sodium-potassium pumps then return the membrane

Table 3-1   Comparison of the Transmission Properties of the Receptive and Transmissive Segments of the Cell

Receptive Segment	Transmissive Segment
Impulse transmission Graded Decremental Passive spread	Impulse transmission All-or-none Nondecremental Self-propagating threshold
Repolarization Postsynaptic enzyme destroys transmitter substance Sodium-potassium pumps	Repolarization Sodium-potassium pumps reestablish concentration-diffusion and voltage gradients
Coding of information Amplitude of postsynaptic potential	Coding of information Discharge frequency

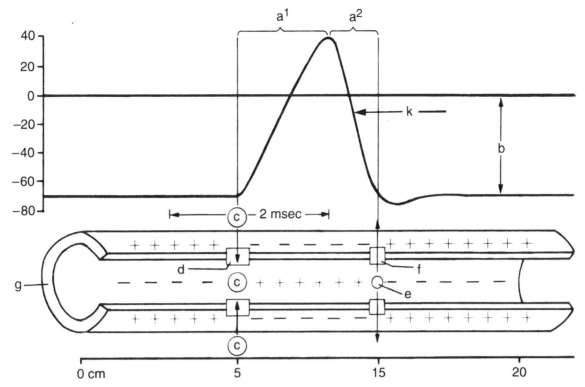

Fig. 3-2

a	*Action potential*
a¹	Relative refractory period
a²	Absolute refractory period
b	Resting membrane potential
c	Sodium
d	Sodium channel
e	Potassium
f	Potassium channel
g	Cell membrane

to its resting state. For temporal summation to be effective in bringing the postsynaptic membrane to threshold, each wave of transmitter substance must reach the postsynaptic membrane before it has recovered from the effects of previous transmitter substance. By doing so, the depolarizing effects of the transmitter substance will be added to the membrane potential encountered on arrival and will progressively, in a step-like fashion, drive the postsynaptic membrane to reach threshold. Thus, temporal summation is proportional to amount of transmitter substance released and time between each release.

Spatial summation occurs when two or more synapses affect adjacent segments of the postsynaptic membrane at the same time (Fig. 3-4). The postsynaptic effects of spatial summation accumulate algebraically. If the synapses are of similar physiological type (either excitatory or inhibitory), the postsynaptic effect is summed and becomes greater than the effect of the two occurring individually (Fig. 3-4A). If the synapses are of opposite physiological type and the discharge from each synapse is of equal magnitude, their postsynaptic effects will negate each other (Fig. 3-4B).

The cumulative effects of all synaptic input (temporal and spatial summation) are evaluated at the axon hillock. The axon hillock is located in the initial segment of the axon and acts as a trigger zone because it contains many voltage-gated channels with lower thresholds. If threshold is reached, the axon hillock triggers an action potential, which is then propagated down the entire axon. Because the electrical potential of the receptive segment of the neuron fluctuates continuously in response to the ongoing effects of thousands of synapses (neuronal integration), threshold can be reached repeatedly. Each time threshold is reached, a nerve impulse is generated. Therefore, the integrated effect of all synaptic discharge is encoded as the frequency of nerve impulse generation. The frequency reflects stimulus intensity and is transmitted to other cells in the neural network.

As a result of propagating an action potential, both concentration and voltage gradients are lost. Until the sodium-potassium pumps have restored the resting membrane potential, and thus the two gradients, no further impulse propagation is possible. This condition of nonexcitability (refraction) is called the absolute refractory period and extends from the moment of initiating the action potential to a few milliseconds after it has passed (see Fig. 3-2). As the pumps restore the resting membrane potential and the gradients become regenerated, the absolute refractory period is replaced by a relative refractory period. During this time, additional nerve impulses may be generated. However, to do so, the critical threshold is raised so that more postsynaptic depolarization is required before an action potential is triggered. After the relative refractory period, if no impulses are generated, both the resting membrane potential and normal critical threshold will be restored.

Indirectly Gated Chemical Transmission: Second Messengers

Thus far, discussion of synaptic transmission has dealt exclusively with directly gated chemical effects. This type of neuronal response is fast and short-lived. A second type of chemical synaptic transmission also exists: second messenger gated transmission. Second messengers are produced inside the postsynaptic cell by a complex series of events triggered by the arrival of direct synaptic transmission. After the transmitter substance arrives, the receptors are coupled to enzymes that synthesize second messengers, which then act on ion channels. This type of neuronal response is slow and long-lived. Indirect chemically gated synaptic transmission is slow to develop because of the steps involved in synthesizing second messengers. It is long-lived because second messengers activate a cascade of reactions inside the cell that endure. This type of neuronal response is well adapted to produce or regulate sustained types of behavior. For example, sustained muscular contraction requires the continuous flow of activity across a synapse and is regulated by second messengers.

Electrical Synapses

Information is also transferred between neurons at a second type of synapse: electrical synapses. The cleft at an electrical synapse is extremely small and bridged by channels (gap junctions) that establish direct connection between the cytoplasm of presynaptic and postsynaptic cells (Fig. 3-5). Electrical transmission occurs by current flow directly from one cell to the next. Gap junction channels extend between cells and are permeable to small molecules and some second messengers. Because the transport mechanism is direct, electrical synapses are the fastest form of synaptic communication. Electrical synapses are rare in the human nervous system.

The Location of Synaptic Connections Influences Effectiveness

The closer a synaptic connection is to the axon hillock of the postsynaptic cell, the more influential it is in determining whether threshold is reached. Excitatory synapses tend to be located on the dendrites while inhibitory synapses are usually found on the cell body, making it easier for them to override excitatory synapses. Of course, the cell membrane automatically integrates all synaptic input and threshold at the axon hillock determines whether an action potential will occur.

Axoaxonic synapses occur most frequently on the terminal bouton of the postsynaptic cell. They are designed to modulate the amount of transmitter substance released by the postsynaptic cell. By depolarizing the postsynaptic cell, an axoaxonic synapse causes

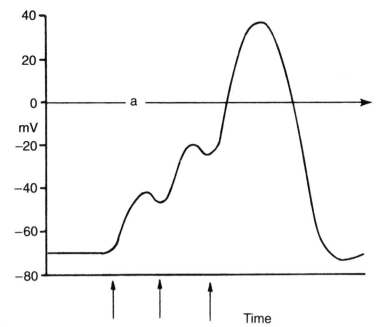

Fig. 3-3

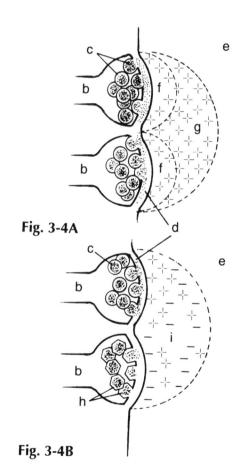

Fig. 3-4A

Fig. 3-4B

a	Temporal summation
b	Terminal bouton
c	Facilitatory synaptic vesicles
d	Transmitter substance
e	Postsynaptic membrane
f	Area affected by single synapse
g	Spatially summated area
h	Inhibitory synaptic vesicles
i	Algebraic cancellation

less transmitter substance to be released, or by hyperpolarizing the postsynaptic cell, it causes more transmitter substance to be released.

Neurophysiology of Single Cells

Neurons generate two types of potentials: synaptic and action. The synaptic or dendritic potential is a local disturbance of the resting state generated in the receptive segment of the cell as the result of neurotransmitter interacting with the cell membrane. Synaptic potentials are localized, nonpropagated, graded fluctuations of the resting membrane potential and can be excitatory (EPSP) when the neurotransmitter causes depolarization of the cell membrane or inhibitory (IPSP) when the neurotransmitter causes hyperpolarization of the cell membrane. Synaptic potentials are usually short (15–20 msec) and they do not have a refractory period.

Action potentials usually arise from the axon hillock and propagate along the axon. (In the case of first-order neurons, they can also arise from the dendrite.) An action potential occurs only when the neuronal membrane is depolarized beyond a critical (threshold) level. The spike discharge is brief (usually less than 1 msec). It is an all-or-none phenomenon propagated the length of the axon and followed by a temporary period of refraction.

Neurophysiology of Neuronal Networks

Neurons in the central nervous system do not function in isolation but participate as one part of a functional system or neural network. Neurons within the functional system have rich synaptic interconnections and the electrical activity within that system reflects the summed effects of all the dendritic and action potentials occurring within the system. Often, the output of a functional system is the control of a particular type of behavior. Changes in that behavior are produced by and reflect the changing aggregate activity within its control system. For example, movement is the behavioral output of thousands of neurons spontaneously orchestrated by the motor control system to accomplish a specific movement goal.

Clinical Aspects

Some clinical aspects of excitation, conduction, and transmission deal with transient or rapidly reversible abnormalities. Transient abnormalities in the physiology of neurons cause transient symptoms and signs and may produce no permanent damage to the cells. Interference with neuronal function can occur in two ways: by altering membrane conductance or by changing ionic concentrations. Some interference occurs along the axon. Local anesthesia, for example, acts on the axon to prevent changes in sodium conductance, thereby blocking the conduction of action potentials. However, most interference occurs at the synaptic junction.

Chemical synapses are designed to produce and respond to drug interactions, which makes them particularly susceptible to "other drug interactions." Some drugs act by blocking transmitter release and others act by blocking transmitter uptake. For example, benzodiazepines and barbiturates both bind to receptor sites for inhibitory transmitters and enhance the chloride flux through these channels, thereby hyperpolarizing the membrane and making it more difficult for the neuron to reach threshold and discharge. The opiate family of drugs produce analgesia by blocking the uptake of transmitter on second-order neurons in the central pain pathway.

Abnormal ionic concentrations, both intracellular and extracellular, may affect neuronal function. Both abnormally low and abnormally high ionic concentrations impede neuronal function and the behavior controlled by those neurons. Decreased extracellular potassium (hypokalemia) hyperpolarizes the cell membrane. Increased extracellular potassium (hyperkalemia), as seen in kidney disease, depolarizes the cell membrane, with possible neuronal hyperactivity, anoxia, fainting, and seizures. Decreased calcium (hypocalcemia) can block synaptic transmission by blocking the release of transmitter substance.

Disruption of excitation, conduction, and transmission is also the mechanism of some disease processes and lethal poisons. Myasthenia gravis is an autoimmune disease in which antibodies are produced against acetylcholine (ACh) receptors in muscle. The muscular weakness that results can be reversed by drugs that inhibit acetylcholinesterase, the enzyme that degrades ACh. Curare produces its muscle-paralyzing effects with a similar ACh uptake blocking mechanism. The most poisonous snakes and electric eels inject neurotoxins that bind irreversibly to ACh receptor sites blocking any further uptake. Botulism, a potentially lethal form of food poisoning, produces its effects by a presynaptic block of ACh release as its mechanism of effectiveness. Multiple sclerosis (MS) is caused by a demyelinating lesion of the axon that disrupts transmission and produces weakness and sensory loss.

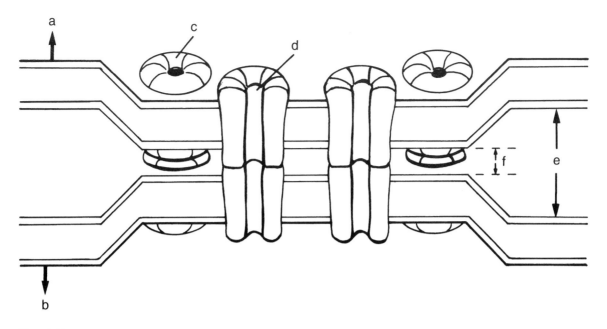

Fig. 3-5

a	Presynaptic cytoplasm
b	Postsynaptic cytoplasm
c	Channel protein
d	Channel formed by pores in each membrane
e	Chemical synaptic cleft
f	Electrical synaptic cleft (gap junction)

4 Development and Growth of the Nervous System

Overview

Unlike most cells in the human body that are replaced on a regular basis, the neurons developed by early postnatal life must last a lifetime since they are never replaced. Luckily for us, however, the specific connections between these neurons can change throughout life as a result of experience; therefore, we can continue to learn and acquire new functional abilities if we so desire. Behind the cardiovascular system, the nervous system is the second organ system to become formed and functional.

The basic framework of the mature nervous system, including the general pattern of connections between most cells, is formed and functional by the end of the fourth week of gestation. The location of the structures in the mature nervous system is determined by the orderly development in the primitive nervous system. The entire nervous system develops from the neural plate. The neural tube forms the central nervous system, the brain and spinal cord, and the neural crests form important components of the peripheral nervous system. Development of the individual (ontogenesis) includes a replication of evolutionary development (phylogenesis) of the nervous system so that older systems develop first, whereas newer systems are not yet developed fully, even at birth. Once a structure is developed in the vertebrate brain, it usually remains, and if new structures evolve they are added to the outside of the system in addition to the older structures. This phylogenic development has produced a human brain in which the old life-support systems (reticular formation) are buried deep in the core (sometimes referred to as the inner tube) while the newer, higher-order functioning systems (cerebral cortex and corticospinal tract) are located on the surface.

Disorders of neurodevelopment may occur at any developmental stage. The results of such disorders determine the developmental process that was disrupted. Most common neurodevelopment disorders are failure of the neural tube to close properly and failures of cell proliferation and migration.

Origin of the Nervous System

The formation of the neural tube begins on the 18th day of gestation. By this time of embryonic development, the early stage of two-layer development (gastrulation) is complete. Transformation from a two-layer to a three-layer embryo is achieved by the outgrowth of the mesoderm from the midline primitive streak into the area between the two layers. The notochord, a column of specialized mesodermal cells, grows forward from the anterior end of the primitive streak (Hensen's node, Fig. 4-1A). The ectoderm overlying the notochord is induced to form the neural plate. This plate is exposed to both the surface dorsally and the amniotic fluid ventrally. Skin will develop from the adjacent ectodermal tissue. Certain portions of the ectoderm differentiate and thicken in the head region to form placodes (progenitors of special sense organs), such as the eyes (optic placode), ears (auditory placode), and nose (nasal placode). The neural plate enlarges and its lateral edges are raised to form two longitudinally oriented neural ridges. These ridges continue to grow medially, creating a groove that continues to deepen (Fig. 4-1B) until the ridges meet and unite in the midline to form the neural tube (Fig. 4-1C). This midline union begins in the cervical region and progresses both rostrally and caudally until the entire plate becomes the enclosed neural tube by the 25th day. Thus, the neural tube was formed in approximately one week, the 18th to the 25th day. After closure, the neural tube detaches from the skin and migrates below the surface. Basically, the nervous system originates as a superficial structure and then migrates beneath the body surface.

When the neural tube migrates below the surface, two columns of cells at the junction of the skin ectoderm and neuroectoderm detach from the neural tube and form the neural crest (Fig 4-1C). Neural crest cells are the progenitors of most of the peripheral nervous system, forming both neural and nonneural cells: neurons of all sensory, autonomic, and enteric ganglia (controlling the intestines); neurilemma (Schwann) cells and satellite cells of the ganglia; cells of the pia mater and arachnoid (protective coverings of the brain; see Chap. 5) as well as the sclera and choroid of the eye; cells of the adrenal medulla; and receptor cells in the carotid body (help to regulate blood oxygen concentration and pressure).

Differentiation of Neurons and Glial Cells

During the peak of cell development, the embryonic neural tube contains four concentric zones: ventricular, subventricular, intermediate, and marginal. The ventricular zone is the region of highest mitotic activity. Ventricular cells are the progenitors of neurons and macroglia (astroglia and oligodendroglia) of the central nervous system. The subventricular zone is composed of smaller cells undergoing mitosis. This zone persists only a few days in the spinal cord but years in the brain. The neurons and macroglia produced here form the rhombic lips located on the lateral margins of the medulla and the ganglionic eminence located in the floor of each lateral ventricle. The rhombic lips generate brain stem and cerebellar neurons, including the billions of interneurons of the cerebellar cortex.

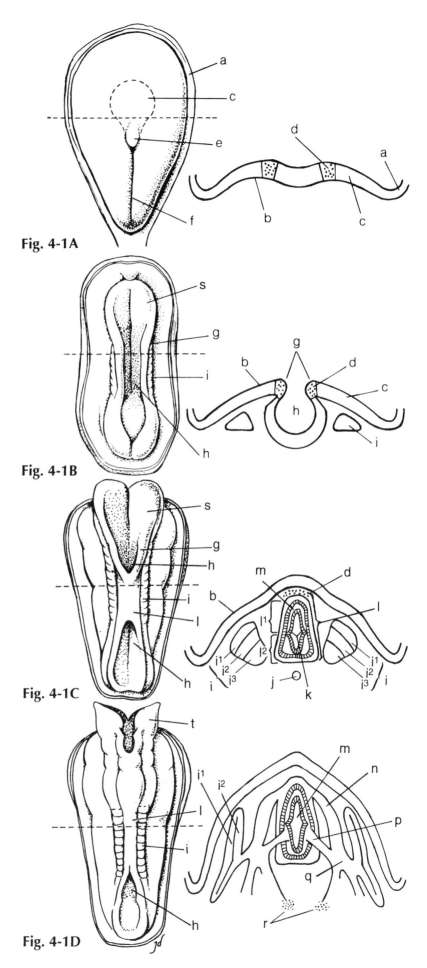

a	Amnion
b	Ectoderm
c	Neural plate
d	Neural crest
e	Hensen's node
f	Primitive streak
g	Neural ridge
h	Neural groove
i	Somite
i^1	Dermatome
i^2	Myotome
i^3	Sclerotome
j	Notochord
k	Sulcus limitans
l	Neural tube
l^1	Alar plate
l^2	Basal plate
m	Central canal
n	Dorsal root
p	Ventral root
q	Spinal nerve
r	Sympathetic ganglion
s	Brain plate
t	Brain

Fig. 4-1A

Fig. 4-1B

Fig. 4-1C

Fig. 4-1D

The ganglionic eminence generates many of the small neurons of the basal ganglia and other telencephalic nuclei. After mitotic activity ceases, cells migrate from the ventricular and subventricular zones to the intermediate zone or further to form the cortical plates. As a rule, larger neurons differentiate first and become transmission type neurons and small neurons differentiate later and become local interneurons. The intermediate (mantle) zone develops into the gray matter in the nervous system including the cortex of cerebrum and cerebellum (most of the cells of the cerebellar cortex are derived from the rhombic lips). The marginal zone develops into the white matter consisting primarily of myelinated and unmyelinated axons and macroglia.

Synaptogenesis

Before the developing neurons of the nervous system can be organized into functional units, they must communicate with one another. It is estimated that the trillion neurons in the nervous system form one hundred trillion synaptic connections. The basic mechanism by which neurons "know" where to migrate and with whom to form synaptic connections is a combination of gene expression and cell-to-cell interactions. The current understanding of how neurons are guided to their final destination and establish synaptic connections with target neurons is a modification of the chemoaffinity hypothesis. Maturing neurons and their axons respond to diffusible chemotrophic molecules that establish chemical attractions from target cells. These molecules attract migrating neurons along designated routes to their final locations and guide the developing axons to their destination to form synaptic connections. The navigation of axonal growth is directed by the growth cone at its tip. Specific proteins on the surface of the growth cone respond to chemotrophic signals of certain molecules in order to guide the developing axon along its proper path past some cells en route to its target cell.

The formation of a synapse, including the location on the postsynaptic cell, type of neurotransmitter, number of receptor sites on the postsynaptic membrane, and other specific details, is determined by an interaction between presynaptic and postsynaptic cells. Once formed, a synapse may be modified by environmental influences. Most synaptic connections are established at an early stage of development. Early synaptic connections follow genetically stereotypical patterns including the specific locations of the target cell. As the neuron becomes electrically active and is integrated into a functional network, some synapses remain and others are retracted. In general, a framework of structure and connections within the nervous system is worked out in two steps. First, during earlier stages of development, an oversupply of neurons and synaptic connections is produced; during later stages of growth, a functional reorganization and selective culling of nonessential elements takes place. This general framework then undergoes a constant activity-dependent physiological reorganization ("fine tuning") to develop and refine the neural control systems necessary to meet the current functional demands of the individual.

It is current theory that by birth most of the nervous system is prewired but a significant portion remains capable of changing. By maturation, structural connections that were originally more plastic are thought to become "hard wired." The synaptic changes that underlie learning are believed to be physiological, that is, a "reweighting" of synaptic influence, rather than the formation of new structural connections.

Following neuronal injury, some synaptic connections may die and the vacant position on the postsynaptic neuron is usually filled by the formation of new synaptic connections. Reestablishment of synaptic connections following injury is thought to be one possible mechanism underlying the recovery of function following neuronal damage. For a complete discussion of recovery of function, see the clinical aspects section of Chap. 2, The Neuron.

The Peripheral Nervous System

As the neural tube closes, the mesoderm lateral to the tube becomes segregated into paired cell masses called somites (Fig. 4-1C). Somites differentiate into three components: the sclerotome, myotome, and dermatome. The sclerotome is located ventromedial in the somite and differentiates into the bony covering of the central nervous system: the cartilage and bone of the vertebral column and base of the skull. The remnant of the notochord becomes engulfed by the sclerotome and forms the nucleus pulposus of the intervertebral disk. The myotome is located in the intermediate portion of the somite and differentiates into the striated skeletal muscle of the body, except the muscles of the head and neck, which are derived from the branchial arches. The dermatome is located lateral in the somite and differentiates into the dermis, the connective tissue layer of the skin.

The 31 pairs of somites are arranged in sequence from the first cervical through the last coccygeal level (Fig. 4-1C). Each somite receives its innervation from adjacent segments of the neural crest and neural tube (Fig. 4-1D). Bipolar neural crest cells become first-order sensory neurons, with their cell bodies located in the dorsal root ganglion, distal segment innervating sensory receptors in the somite, and proximal segment synapsing in the alar plate. Motor neurons have their cell bodies located in the basal plate and axons innervate effector organs (muscles or glands) in the somite. Sensory and motor fibers to each somite unite to form a single spinal nerve. The 31 pairs of somites become innervated by 31 pairs of spinal nerves, thus forming the sclerotomal, myotomal, and dermatomal innervation patterns seen in the mature nervous system (see Fig. 6-5).

An axon has its full complement of neurilemma cells by the time it innervates an end organ (sensory

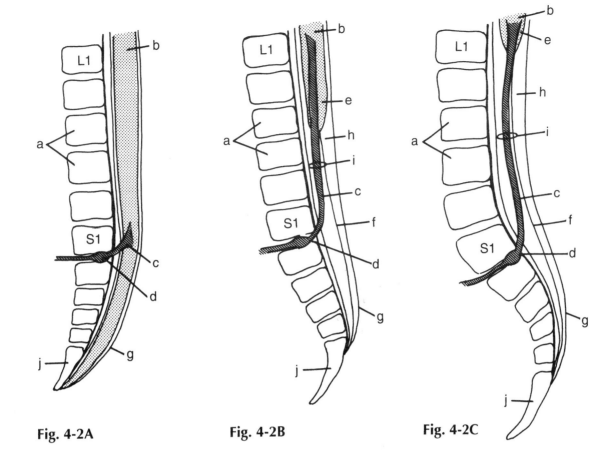

Fig. 4-2A   **Fig. 4-2B**   **Fig. 4-2C**

a	Vertebral bodies
b	Spinal cord
c	First sacral dorsal root
d	Dorsal root ganglion
e	Conus medullaris
f	Filum terminale
g	Dura mater
h	Lumbar cistern
i	Cauda equina
j	Coccyx

or motor). Myelination begins early in the second trimester and continues into early adult life. The period of most rapid myelination occurs between the third trimester and two years of age. This corresponds to the period of most rapid brain growth and physiological maturation. The myelination of tracts and regions of the central nervous system follows a well-defined and orderly progression. The progression of myelination correlates highly with the progression of physiological maturation and development of specific functions and skills. For example, in the corticospinal tract, myelination begins at about the 36th week of gestation and progresses sequentially throughout the spinal cord by about age two. Myelination correlates well with the acquisition of motor skills: earlier in the cervical regions correlating with head control, then in the upper extremities correlating with independent limb manipulation, and later in the lower extremities correlating with standing, walking, and running.

Myelination begins when the axon reaches 1 to 2 micrometers (µm) in diameter. During the subsequent growth in length, the internode (the area covered by neurilemma cells) elongates. Myelination can be considered to be synonymous with neuronal development. Two generalized developmental patterns exist within the nervous system: Myelination occurs first in the axons that mature to the largest diameter, and within the sensory systems, maturation progresses from distal to proximal with the more rostral levels developing last.

The precise mechanisms responsible for organizing the peripheral nervous system into complex patterns, which are basically similar among individuals, are not clearly understood. However, some generalizations are possible. The outgrowths from the basal plate and neural crest occur early in development and innervate the adjacent somites. As the somites differentiate and their subdivisions migrate to their respective locations in the body, they maintain their connections with nerve fibers. Thus, the elongating nerve process is "towed" out to the periphery by the developing nonneural tissue such as muscle cells. These original nerve fibers then provide the "path" along which subsequent nerve fibers grow to form peripheral nerves. Growth occurs at the tip of the nerve filament after a nerve growth factor is projected from the peripheral end and follows the path of the original filament. Neurilemma cells accompany the growth process, and subsequently myelination occurs. An example of the consequences of the towing of nerve fibers by the primordial muscle cells is found in the innervation of the leg muscles. Muscles located as far apart as the hip and ankle receive their innervation from the same segmental level of the spinal cord. The gluteus maximus is derived from somites of the fifth lumbar and first and second sacral segments. After these somites are innervated, the primordial muscle cells begin to migrate and tow their innervation with them to their final destination in the hip girdle. Other portions of the same somites migrate fur-

ther down the leg. Hence, some fibers of the fifth lumbar and first and second sacral nerves innervate the gluteus maximus via the inferior gluteal nerve, and other fibers innervate muscles of the lower leg and foot through long branches of the sciatic nerve.

A reciprocal relationship exists between peripheral nerves and peripheral tissue. For example, a muscle cell that has not yet been innervated is receptive to becoming innervated. However, once innervated, the same cells accept no other functional connections. This mechanism helps to ensure that all muscle fibers become innervated but restricts the number of innervations so as to promote good muscle control. Nerve fibers possess the ability to branch, so that several uninnervated muscle fibers may become innervated by a single axon. This potential is retained throughout life, as is the potential of a nerve fiber to grow in length. Nerve regeneration and collateral branching are mechanisms that underlie the recovery of function following damage to the nervous system. The peripheral nervous system differs from the central nervous system in this regard. For a complete discussion of these issues, see Chap. 2, The Neuron.

The Spinal Cord

A longitudinal groove (sulcus limitans) extends along either side of the inner surface of the neural tube, dividing it into alar and basal plates. The portion of the neural tube dorsal to the sulcus limitans is the alar plate, which forms the sensory region of the spinal cord and brain stem. The gray matter in this region differentiates into nuclei that are associated with the sensory input from peripheral, spinal, and cranial nerves. The portion of the neural tube ventral to the sulcus limitans is the basal plate, which differentiates into the motor nuclei of spinal and cranial nerves. The gray matter in this region is made up of the cell bodies of efferent neurons, which innervate peripheral effector mechanisms (muscles and glands). Also, the structures that develop from the tissue closer to the central canal (inner tube) form the sensory and motor neurons of the phylogenetically older visceral nervous system, which is concerned with the control of internal organs and homeostasis. The structures that develop from the tissue closer to the perimeter (outer tube) form the sensory and motor neurons of the phylogenetically newer somatic nervous system (somatic because it is derived from somites), which is concerned with sensing exteroceptive information of moving the body.

Up to about the third fetal month, the spinal cord extends the entire length of the developing vertebral column (Fig. 4-2A). At the time, the dorsal (sensory) and ventral (motor) roots of the spinal nerves extend laterally outward at right angles to the spinal cord. The roots unite in the intervertebral foramina to form the spinal nerves. Because the vertebral column grows faster than the spinal cord, after the third fetal month, the spinal cord no longer extends the entire length of the vertebral column. At birth, the caudal end of the

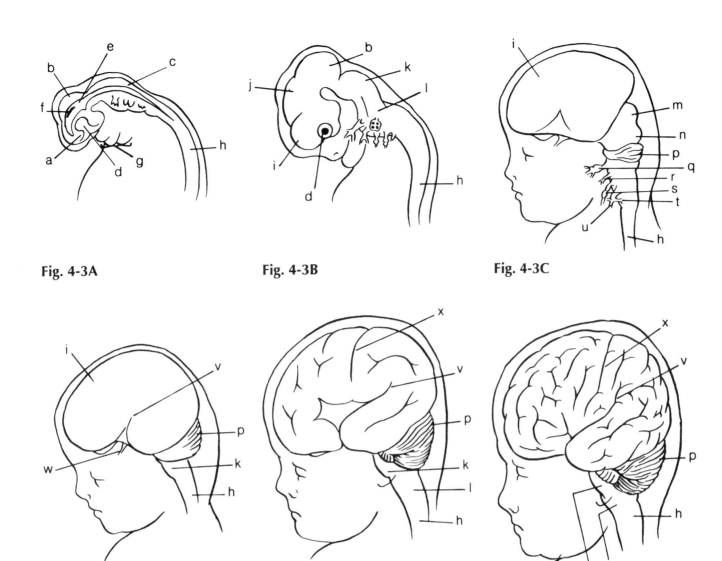

Fig. 4-3A   Fig. 4-3B   Fig. 4-3C

Fig. 4-3D   Fig. 4-3E   Fig. 4-3F

a	Prosencephalon	m	Superior colliculus
b	Mesencephalon	n	Inferior colliculus
c	Rhombencephalon	p	Cerebellum
d	Optic placode	q	Trigeminal nerve (V)
e	Ventricular system	r	Facial nerve (VII)
f	Choroid plexus	s	Glossopharyngeal nerve (IX)
g	Branchiomeric arches	t	Hypoglossal nerve (XII)
h	Spinal cord	u	Vagus nerve (X)
i	Telencephalon	v	Lateral fissure
j	Diencephalon	w	Optic nerve (II)
k	Metencephalon	x	Central sulcus
l	Myelencephalon		

spinal cord (conus medullaris) is located at the level of the L3 vertebra (Fig. 4-2B). In the adult the conus medullaris is located approximately between the L1 and L2 vertebrae (Fig. 4-2C). During the long period of differential growth of the spinal cord and vertebral column, the nerve root filaments between the conus medullaris and intervertebral foramina become elongated. As a result of this disparity in growth rate, the lumbar, sacral, and coccygeal nerve roots become directed caudally at an acute angle to the spinal cord. The bundle of elongated nerve fibers that is located within the vertebral canal caudal to the conus medullaris is termed the cauda equina (horse's tail). The area below the L2 vertebra that contains the cauda equina is the safest place to perform a spinal tap in order to remove cerebrospinal fluid. A needle inserted in this area will simply move the nerve fibers of the cauda equina aside without damaging them. Accompanying the cauda equina is the nonneural filum terminale, which anchors the caudal end of the spinal cord by attaching to the dorsal surface of the second coccygeal vertebra (Fig. 4-2B, C).

As the longitudinal differentiation of the neural tube continues it is helpful to keep in mind the general principles that govern the location of functional systems. Sensory systems are derived from the alar plate and motor systems are derived from the basal plate. Visceral systems are derived from the inner tube and somatic systems are derived from the outer tube.

The Brain

Prenatal Development

At the end of the fourth week of gestation, there are three enlargements at the rostral end of the neural tube (Fig. 4-3A). These dilations are the three primary subdivisions of the brain: the hindbrain (rhombencephalon), midbrain (mesencephalon), and forebrain (prosencephalon). The central canal of the neural tube has dilated into the rudimentary ventricular system of the brain. In the thin roof of the ventricles, the choroid plexus develops and produces cerebrospinal fluid.

By the end of the sixth week, significant brain development has taken place (Fig. 4-3B). The rhombencephalon has divided into the myelencephalon (the future medulla) and the metencephalon (the future pons and cerebellum). The mesencephalon remains undivided as the midbrain. The prosencephalon has divided into the diencephalon (the future thalamic complex and third ventricle) and the telencephalon (the future cerebral hemispheres, basal ganglia, and lateral ventricles). With continued development of the brain, individual structures will become differentiated. Although it is presently unclear whether any new nerve cells are produced after birth, it is quite evident that almost all nerve cell production is completed during prenatal life.

The sequential development of the brain from the 11-week-old embryo to the newborn is seen in Fig. 4-3C to F. By the 11th week of gestation, the essential form of the brain may be seen although the external surface is still smooth. Fissures begin to form around the fourth month of gestation, with the lateral fissures occurring first followed by the posterolateral sulcus of the cerebellum, central sulcus, calcarine sulcus, and parietooccipital sulcus by the fifth month. The main sulci and gyri of the cerebral cortex are present by the seventh month. In the newborn, cortical development is far from complete. The smaller sulci and gyri are not yet formed, differentiation of gray and white matter is poor, the pia mater is loosely attached, and the blood supply is not yet fully formed.

Postnatal Development

Development of the brain continues, at a progressively slower pace, until approximately age 10. The critical period of postnatal brain growth is from birth to about two years, by which age the relative size and proportions of the brain and its subdivisions are essentially similar to those of the adult brain. Myelination, the neurodevelopmental equivalent of maturation, is complete by this time. Also, all sulci and gyri have developed, the gray matter has differentiated from the white matter, and the cortical blood supply is fully developed. As with the development of other physiological systems, the brain of a girl develops more rapidly than that of a boy up to about age three; however, by puberty the brains of boys outweigh those of girls (1,375 g vs. 1,250 g, respectively). At birth, the brain is disproportionately large for the body (10% of the body weight of the newborn but only 2% of the mature adult). From birth to adulthood the body grows faster than the brain. The brain appears to retain its ability to change and adapt throughout life; as with other functional systems, this ability seems to decline progressively with age. In the absence of pathology, the slope of age-related changes appears to be activity dependent, as in the saying "use it or lose it!"

Aging of the Brain During Postnatal Life

In the absence of pathology, the brain loses approximately 10 percent of its weight between the ages of 20 and 90. Weight loss is due to a progressive decline in the number of neurons because as neurons die they are not replaced. As the cortex loses cells, the gyri become more narrow and the sulci become broader. The loss of cells is not uniform in all regions but affects the cortex more than the brain stem. Within the cortex, the neocortex is most affected, particularly in the frontal lobe, including precentral gyrus, primary visual cortex, and cingulate gyrus. The functional changes with age include a 20 percent decrease in cerebral blood supply, a 10 percent decrease in conduction velocity, and a general increase in sensory threshold such that higher stimulus intensity is required to produce a response, including a reflex response. Contributing to this increase may be the decrease in the number of sensory receptors (taste buds and rods and cones) and a decrease in the number of fibers in large nerves.

Age-related changes also occur within the neuron.

The cell body loses Nissl substance and may accumulate useless material including organelles and pigment. Aging of the neuron is seen by a change in size (either increase or decrease). The quantity of essential proteins tends to increase progressively from birth to age 40, remains stable from 40 to 60, and decreases from 60 years on. Changes also occur in nonneural tissue including the protective covering of the brain (meninges), which becomes more calcified and rigid.

Clinical Aspects

Essentially, neurodevelopment occurs in six stages. However, some of the stages occur simultaneously. The stages are named for the developmental process that is dominant at that time. Disorders of neurodevelopment may occur at any stage. Such disorders are generally classified according to the dominant process occurring at the time they arise. Most common are failures of the neural tube to close properly and failures of cell proliferation and migration.

Stage one is formation of the neural tube. This process dominates the third and fourth weeks of gestation. Disorders occurring at this time involve failure of the neural tube to close. The general class of failure to close caudally is often referred to as spina bifida. Listed in order of severity, these disorders include spina bifida occulta, a defect involving only the vertebral arch; meningocele, protrusion of the meninges through the bony deficit into a sac (cele); meningomyelocele, inclusion of herniated spinal cord into the cele; and myeloschisis, in which the spinal cord is completely open to the surface through a failure of the bone or skin to close. The same disorder may produce malformations at the rostral end of the neural tube. Listed in order of severity, they include cranium bifidum, cranial meningocele, meningoencephalocele, cranioschisis (anencephaly), and craniorachischisis, in which the neural tube is completely open to the surface.

Stage two is formation of the telencephalon and closure of the branchial arches. This stage dominates the fifth and sixth weeks of gestation. The branchial arches close anteriorly and failure to close produces craniofacial deformities (e.g., cleft palate). Defects produced during this stage may also cause failure to form the forebrain (holoprosencephaly).

Stage three is proliferation of cells in the ventricular and subventricular zones. This process is most active from the 8th to 16th week of gestation. Genetic, chemical, or infectious disturbances of the proliferating neuroblasts may result in an insufficient number of neurons to form a normal-sized brain (microencephaly). Defective proliferation may be manifest in the number or type of synapses formed between neurons, which may account for some cases of mental retardation in grossly normally structured brains.

Stage four is the active migration of neurons and spongioblasts (cells that form the meninges). This process is most active from the 12th to the 20th week of gestation. Disturbance of development at this time causes collections of neurons or other gray matter components where they do not belong (heterotopia). Disturbance may produce abnormally large gyri (pachygyria) or abnormally small gyri (microgyria). Disorders of migration may be either localized or generalized, and they often occur along with disorders of proliferation because the two stages overlap in time.

Stage five is cell differentiation and is most active from the sixth month of gestation to maturity. At this time cells are growing in size, forming synaptic connections, and developing neurochemical transmitters. Disruption during this stage does not generally lead to gross anatomical deformity, but rather to functional disturbances such as learning disabilities and mental retardation.

Stage six is myelination of the nervous system. This stage extends from the last half of gestation through age 18 but is most active from birth through age 2. Disruption of myelination does not produce obvious structural malformation. Failure of myelination produces loss of the function controlled by those neurons. Failure of myelination due to genetic disorders (leukodystrophies) usually occurs in the first two years of life.

Malnutrition during fetal life, infancy, and childhood has deleterious effects on neurodevelopment. The result of extreme nutritional deficiencies that occur during the critical developmental period is irreversible brain damage. The critical period extends from the second trimester of gestation through age one. Maternal protein malnutrition reduces the rate of proliferation of new neurons and glial cells in the fetus. Even if the child is fed a nutritionally adequate diet after the critical period, the damage cannot be completely reversed. These children exhibit a 10 to 20 percent decrease in IQ, decreased attention span, transient apathy, lethargy, or hyperirritability. Malnutrition after the critical neurodevelopmental period, even if severe, has no long-term effects on brain function.

5 The Central Nervous System

Overview

The central nervous system consists of the brain and spinal cord, and is responsible for receiving sensory information, determining its meaning, and formulating and initiating adaptive responses in order to accomplish a goal. The central nervous system consists of six main parts: the spinal cord, medulla, pons (and cerebellum), midbrain, diencephalon, and cerebral hemispheres. The spinal cord is directly responsible for controlling the sensory and motor functions of the head and body. The medulla controls life-support functions, including breathing, heart rate, digestion, and arousal. The pons helps to control the cerebellum, which is involved in motor control and motor learning. The midbrain plays an important role in coordinating eye movement. The diencephalon is the primary subcortical sensory integration station and the cerebral hemispheres are the highest level of the central nervous system, controlling cognition, memory, language, motor control, and sensory perception.

The Central Nervous System Consists of Six Main Regions

The six anatomically distinct regions of the mature central nervous system are (1) the spinal cord, (2) the medulla, (3) the pons and cerebellum, (4) the midbrain, (5) the diencephalon, and (6) the cerebral hemispheres (Fig. 5-1).

The Spinal Cord

The spinal cord is the simplest and most caudal portion of the central nervous system. It is responsible for transmitting ascending and descending information and also controls simple behaviors such as reflexes and locomotion under certain circumstances. It is located in the central canal of the vertebral column and, in the mature adult, extends from the base of the skull to the first lumbar vertebra, where it terminates as the conus medullaris (Fig. 5-1). Thus, the spinal cord does not run the entire length of the vertebral column. Beyond the conus medullaris, sensory and motor roots of the lower lumbar, sacral, and coccygeal spinal nerves continue as the cauda equina. The caudal end of the spinal cord is anchored to the vertebral column by the filum terminale, a continuation of the meninges. The spinal cord receives sensory information from the skin, joints, and muscles of the body and contains the cell bodies of motor neurons that innervate skeletal muscle. The spinal cord also receives sensory information from the visceral organs of the body and contains the cell body of preganglionic autonomic fibers that produce reflex response in smooth muscle and glands.

The spinal cord is roughly cylindrical in shape, tapers from rostral to caudal, and is organized along both segmental and longitudinal axes. The 31 pairs of spinal nerves (8 cervical, 12 thoracic, 5 lumbar, 5 sacral, and 1 coccygeal) are oriented along the horizontal or segmental axis. Each segment of the spinal cord gives rise to a pair of spinal nerves that exit the vertebral column from between adjacent vertebrae (intervertebral foramen). Spinal nerves become peripheral nerves by the union of the dorsal and ventral roots. The dorsal roots consist of first-order sensory neurons that arise from sensory receptors, both somatic and visceral. They convey sensory information about conditions in the periphery. The ventral roots consist of motor neurons that innervate muscles and glands. They deliver commands from the central nervous system to the effector organs.

Within the spinal cord there is an orderly arrangement of sensory and motor components. The dorsal portion of the spinal cord is primarily sensory and the ventral portion is mainly motor. The spinal cord contains both gray matter and white matter. The gray matter, which consists of the receptive segment of neurons and glial cells, is located centrally in an "H-like" configuration. The stems of the "H" are located on either side of the spinal cord and consist of dorsal (posterior) and ventral (anterior) horns. The dorsal horn contains sensory nuclei where first-order somatosensory neurons synapse with second-order neurons that project to the brain stem and thalamus. The ventral horn contains motor nuclei that consist of the cell bodies of lower motor neurons that innervate skeletal muscles (dorsolateral and ventromedial cell groups). The intermediate zone separates the dorsal and ventral horns, and contains interneurons that project from the dorsal horn to the ventral horn, project between the nuclei in the ventral horn, and project short and intermediate distances between spinal segments. In the thoracic and upper lumbar segments, this zone also contains the cell bodies of preganglionic sympathetic neurons (lateral horn) and neurons that relay information about the position and movement of the leg and lower trunk directly to the cerebellum (Clarke's column). The stems of the "H" are connected by the gray matter that surrounds the central canal.

On the basis of cytoarchitectural differences, the gray matter has been subdivided into 10 layers (laminae of Rexed, Fig. 5-2B). Outside the first lamina is the dorsal root entry zone. Here, before entering the spinal cord, first-order neurons are arranged by fiber diameter, with large-diameter fibers entering medially and small-diameter fibers entering laterally. Laminae I to VI correspond to the dorsal horn, lamina VII roughly corresponds to the intermediate zone, and laminae VIII

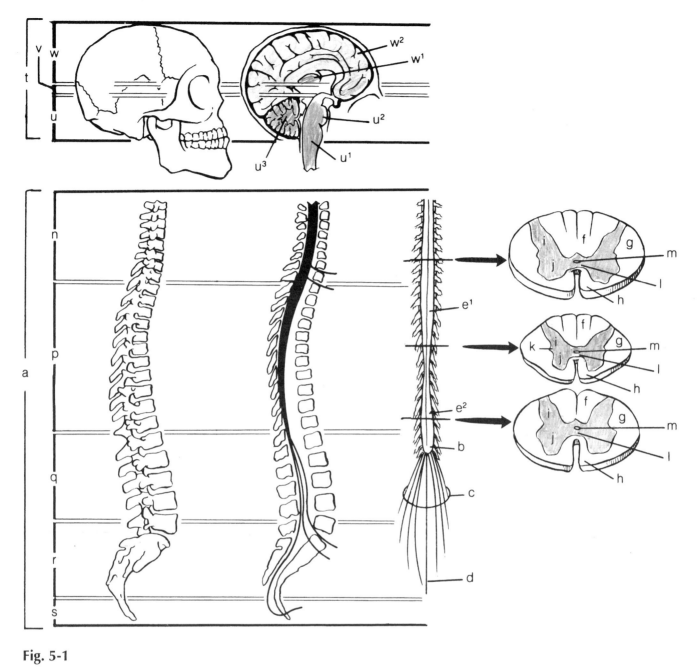

Fig. 5-1

a	*Spinal cord*	(i–m)	*Gray matter*	s	Coccygeal
b	Conus medullaris	i	Dorsal horn	t	*Brain*
c	Cauda equina	j	Ventral horn	u	*Hindbrain*
d	Filum terminale	k	Lateral horn	u¹	Medulla oblongata
e	*Enlargements*	l	Gray commissure	u²	Pons
e¹	Cervical	m	Central canal	u³	Cerebellum
e²	Lumbar	(n–s)	*Spinal nerves*	v	Midbrain
(f–h)	*White matter*	n	Cervical	w	*Forebrain*
f	Dorsal funiculus	p	Thoracic	w¹	Diencephalon
g	Lateral funiculus	q	Lumbar	w²	Cerebrum
h	Ventral funiculus	r	Sacral		

and IX correspond to the ventral horn. Lamina X consists of the cells that surround the central canal.

Lamina I is the marginal zone, and is an important relay site for information about pain and temperature. Lamina II, the substantia gelatinosa, integrates information from unmyelinated first-order neurons with thinly myelinated neurons that project to lamina I. Laminae III, IV, V, and VI constitute the nucleus proprius, which integrates information from first-order sensory neurons with descending input from the brain and contains the cell bodies of projection or tract neurons that ascend to the brain stem. Lamina VII is present only in the thoracic and upper lumbar segments. It contains the cells of Clarke's column (nucleus dorsalis), which relays proprioceptive information from the lower extremity and trunk to the cerebellum, as well as the cell bodies of preganglionic sympathetic fibers, referred to as the lateral horn. Lamina VIII contains interneurons that are important in controlling the contraction of skeletal muscles. Lamina IX consists of pools of lower motor neurons, and lamina X, which immediately surrounds the central canal, receives afferent input similar to laminae I and II. Although the mapping of the laminae of Rexed indicates distinct regions, there is a great deal of overlap between adjacent laminae.

The white matter of the spinal cord surrounds the gray matter and consists of myelinated axons organized into bundles of projection axons for functionally specific systems (tracts). The tracts, both ascending and descending, are oriented along the vertical or longitudinal axis of the spinal cord. The white matter is divided into three primary regions (funiculi): dorsal, ventral, and lateral. The dorsal funiculus extends from the dorsal median septum to the dorsal horn and contains ascending tracts. The ventral funiculus extends from the ventral medial fissure to the ventral horn and contains both ascending and descending tracts. The lateral funiculus extends from the dorsal horn to the ventral horn and also contains both ascending and descending tracts.

The shape and internal structure of the spinal cord varies by segmental level. Two enlargements, cervical and lumbar, were produced by the greater number of neurons necessary to serve the upper and lower extremities. In the enlargements, both dorsal and ventral horns are larger to meet the increased sensory and motor needs of the extremities. Clarke's column and the lateral horn exist only in the thoracic and upper lumbar regions. Finally, the proportion of white matter to gray matter decreases progressively from rostral to caudal because motor fibers exit progressively from rostral to caudal and sensory fibers enter progressively from caudal to rostral.

The Brain Stem: Medulla, Pons, and Midbrain

The next three regions of the central nervous system, the medulla, pons and cerebellum, and midbrain, are referred to collectively as the brain stem. The brain stem participates in three broad categories of function.

In the first category, the ascending and descending pathways that connect the cerebral hemispheres and diencephalon with the spinal cord also pass through and are processed in the brain stem. In the second category, the brain stem gives rise to cranial nerves II through XII. The cranial nerves are functionally analogous to the spinal nerves; that is, they serve the sensory, motor, and visceral needs of the face and head. Some of the cranial nerves are concerned with the special senses of seeing, hearing, tasting, and balance. All 12 cranial nerves are considered individually in Chap. 7. The third functional category of the brain stem involves the control of heart rate, respiration, and arousal. This function is exercised through the reticular formation, a network of nuclei and projection systems that extends the entire length of the brain stem near the midline.

The medulla (medulla oblongata or bulb) is the rostral extension of the spinal cord beyond the foramen magnum and extends to the caudal segment of the pons. The ascending and descending pathways of the spinal cord pass through the medulla. The spinothalamic tracts pass directly through almost unchanged but it is in the medulla that the corticospinal fibers and the dorsal columns of the spinal cord cross the midline. The medulla also contains the nuclei of several cranial nerves, parts of the vestibular and olivary nuclear complexes, and the inferior cerebellar peduncle. The majority of the reticular formation, including the centers that control heart rate, blood pressure, respiration, and arousal, are located in the medulla.

The pons is located between the medulla and midbrain. It protrudes from the ventral surface of the brain stem, contains the nuclei of several cranial nerves, and forms the floor of the fourth ventricle and a bridge between the two cerebellar hemispheres (middle cerebellar peduncles). Neurons from the cerebral hemispheres pass through the pons on their way to the cerebellum (superior cerebellar peduncle). The cerebellum is not classified as part of the brain stem but is considered here because of its anatomical and functional association with the pons.

The cerebellum is located beneath the brain and overlies the dorsal aspect of the pons and medulla. It contains several functionally independent lobes covered by transversely oriented folia. The primary function of the cerebellum is to detect and correct errors in movement. Errors are detected by comparing movement commands from the cerebral cortex with movement-produced somatosensory feedback from the spinal cord and information about balance from the vestibular receptors in the inner ear. Errors are corrected by affecting the planning, timing, and coordination of muscular contractions during movement.

The midbrain is the smallest of the six regions of the central nervous system. It contains the nuclei of the three cranial nerves that regulate eye movement (III, IV, VI). Other brain stem nuclei are involved in the control of skeletal muscle (the mesencephalic nucleus of the trigeminal nerve, red nucleus, and substantia nigra).

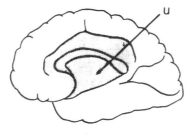

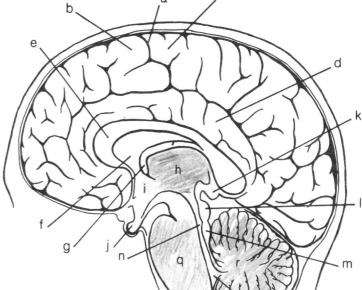

Fig. 5-2A

a	Central sulcus
b	Precentral gyrus
c	Postcentral gyrus
d	Cingulate gyrus
e	Corpus callosum
f	Septum pellucidum
g	Fornix
h	Thalamus
i	Hypothalamus
j	Hypophysis
k	Pineal body
l	Superior colliculus
m	Inferior colliculus
n	Cerebral aqueduct
p	Fourth ventricle
q	Pons
r	Cerebellum
s	Medulla
t	Cervical enlargement
u	Limbic lobe
(I–X)	*Laminae of Rexed*
v	Substantia gelatinosa (II)
w	Nucleus proprius (III, IV, V, and VI)
x	Nucleus dorsalis (VII)
y	Pools of lower motor neurons (IX)

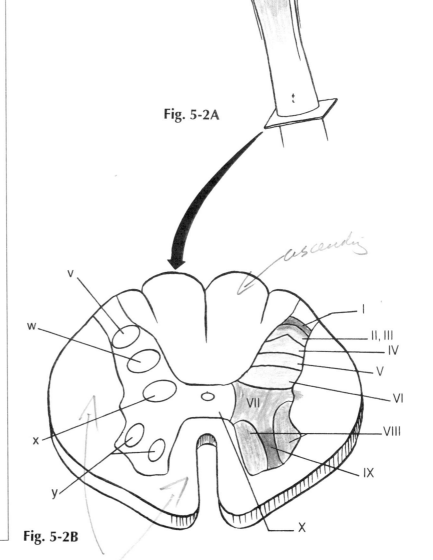

Fig. 5-2B

The Diencephalon

The diencephalon consists of an ovoid mass of gray matter located adjacent to the midline deep within the brain rostral to the midbrain. The third ventricle separates the left half of the diencephalon from the right. The two halves of the diencephalon are often joined by a small mass called the interthalamic adhesion. Each half of the diencephalon can be divided into the thalamus, hypothalamus, subthalamus (which functions as part of the basal ganglia), and epithalamus (Fig. 5-2A).

The thalamus receives, integrates, and distributes almost all sensory and motor information going to the cerebral cortex. As a rule, the thalamus forms reciprocal connections with the cortical region to which it projects. The thalamus is a constellation of nuclei that is divided into three unequal parts by the internal medullary lamina. This band of myelinated fibers separates the medial and lateral masses from the anterior nucleus. Several smaller nuclei are located within the internal medullary lamina near the center of the thalamus. Figure 5-3 is a summary of thalamocortical projections. The medial nuclear mass contains one primary nucleus, the dorsomedial nucleus, which is subdivided into two portions. The small-cell (parvicellular) region has reciprocal connections with the prefrontal cortex that are involved in the sensory integration necessary for abstract thinking and long-term, goal-directed behavior. The large-cell (magnocellular) region has reciprocal connections with the hypothalamus, amygdala, and orbital region of the frontal lobe. The dorsomedial nucleus also has connections with other thalamic nuclei and relays basal ganglia information to the cerebral cortex. The midline nuclei are small and located in the periventricular region and the interthalamic adhesion. They form reciprocal connections with the basal ganglia and limbic system. The lateral nuclear mass is located lateral to the intermedullary lamina and is subdivided into dorsal and ventral tiers of nuclei. The dorsal tier of nuclei are closely related to the association areas of the cerebral cortex and are probably involved in the integration of sensory information. The dorsal tier includes the lateral dorsal nucleus that projects to the cingulate gyrus, the lateral posterior nucleus that projects to the superior parietal lobule, and the pulvinar nucleus that projects to the parietal, temporal, and occipital association cortex. Within the ventral tier of nuclei, the posterior group receive and integrate somatic, visual, auditory, and taste information and transmit the integrated information to the cerebral cortex. The anterior group of ventral tier nuclei receive input from the reticular formation, basal ganglia, cerebellum, and cerebral cortex; process the information; and project to the motor regions of the cerebral cortex.

The hypothalamus is located ventral to the thalamus, forms the floor and ventral walls of the third ventricle, and consists of multiple nuclei. The hypothalamus together with other structures in the limbic system maintains homeostasis through three closely related processes: central control of the visceral nervous system, secretion of hormones, and control of emotional and motivational states. The hypothalamus and limbic system also participate, via the reticular formation, in controlling the level of arousal or general state of awareness.

The subthalamic nucleus is immediately rostral to the midbrain and forms reciprocal connections with the basal ganglia.

The epithalamus is the most dorsal portion of the diencephalon and contains the pineal body, habenular nuclei, and posterior commissure. The pineal body is located on the dorsal surface of the diencephalon in midline rostral to the superior colliculi. It is a nonneural structure consisting exclusively of glial cells (astrocytes). Many postganglionic sympathetic fibers from the superior cervical ganglion terminate here. While the pineal body is involved in the seasonal breeding cycles of other vertebrates, its function remains unknown in humans. The habenular nuclei function as part of the limbic system in controlling drive, motivation, and affect. The posterior commissure is located at the base of the pineal body and contains fibers that cross the midline from one superior colliculus to the other.

The Cerebrum

The cerebral hemispheres are the highest functional level of the brain and by far the largest region of the central nervous system. As seen from a frontal view (Fig. 5-4A), the left and right cerebral hemispheres are separated by a deep vertical crevice (medial longitudinal fissure). Each hemisphere consists of the cerebral cortex, the underlying white matter, and three deeplying nuclei: the basal ganglia, hippocampus, and amygdala (Fig. 5-4B). The cerebral cortex forms the superficial cover of the hemisphere. It appears gray because it consists of unmyelinated cell bodies. The cerebral cortex is continuous across the bottom of major and minor sulci. The white matter consists of the myelinated axons projecting to and from the cortex. These projection fibers form the tightly compressed internal capsule as they pass between the thalamus and basal ganglia. The basal ganglia consist of the caudate nucleus, putamen, globus pallidus, subthalamic nucleus, and substantia nigra and are responsible for initiating and scaling internally generated movements. The hippocampus and amygdala are located in the inferomedial aspect of the hemisphere and function as parts of the limbic system. The hippocampus is involved in the process of memory storage, and the amygdala coordinates autonomic and endocrine responses with changes in emotional states.

The Cerebral Hemisphere is Divided into Five Lobes Concerned with Different Functions

As seen from a frontal view, the brain consists of two cerebral hemispheres. The cerebral cortex is the mantle that covers both cerebral hemispheres and gives them

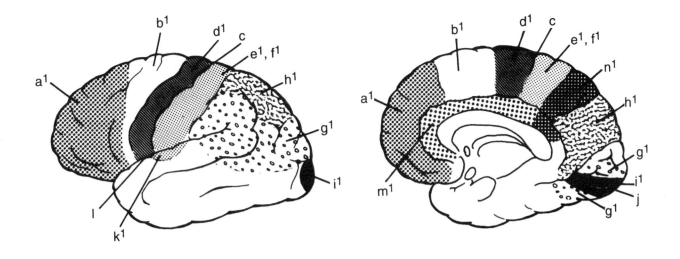

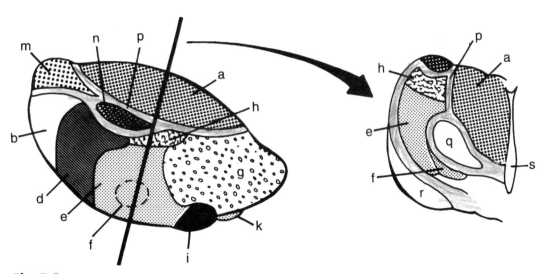

Fig. 5-3

a	Dorsomedial nucleus	i	Lateral geniculate body
a¹	Frontal lobe	i¹	Primary visual cortex
b	Ventral anterior nucleus	j	Calcarine sulcus
b¹	Premotor cortex	k	Medial geniculate body
c	Central sulcus	k¹	Primary auditory cortex
d	Ventral lateral nucleus	l	Lateral sulcus
d¹	Primary motor cortex	m	Anterior thalamic nucleus
e	Ventral posterolateral nucleus	m¹	Cingulate gyrus
e¹	Primary sensory cortex	n	Lateral dorsal nucleus
f	Ventral posteromedial nucleus	n¹	Parietal lobe, medial surface
f¹	Primary sensory cortex	p	Internal medullary lamina
g	Pulvinar	q	Centromedian nucleus
g¹	Parietal temporal occipital cortex	r	Crus cerebri
h	Lateral posterior nucleus	s	Third ventricle
h¹	Parietal lobe		

their convoluted superficial appearance. Some of the convolutions are small and extend for short distances while others are more prominent and remain uninterrupted for long distances. Convolutions are formed by sulci (invaginations) and gyri (mounds) that occurred during development when the rapidly expanding cortex was folded back onto itself repeatedly because of the space limitations imposed by the cranium. The more prominent sulci (sometimes called fissures) serve as superficial landmarks for subdividing the hemisphere into the five lobes: frontal, parietal, temporal, occipital, and limbic (see Fig. 1-2).

The frontal lobe extends from the anterior pole of the brain to the central sulcus (sulcus of Roland). The central sulcus is a prominent sulcus, located at about the middle of the hemisphere, that extends uninterrupted from the medial longitudinal fissure almost to the lateral sulcus (fissure of Sylvius). The parietal lobe extends from the central sulcus to the parietooccipital line. The parietooccipital line parallels a prominent sulcus (parietooccipital sulcus) located on the medial surface of the hemisphere. The occipital lobe extends from the parietooccipital line to the posterior pole of the brain. The temporal lobe lies below the lateral sulcus and rostral to the parietooccipital line. The fifth lobe, the limbic lobe, is seen on the medial aspect of the hemisphere and consists of a ring of structures including the cingulate gyrus and hippocampal formation as well as subcallosal nucleus and several other nuclei along with their interrelated projection fibers (see Fig. 1-2). As seen in this medial view of the hemisphere, the cerebral cortex continues onto the medial surface of the frontal, parietal, temporal, and occipital lobes.

The lobes can be subdivided into primary, secondary, and tertiary projection regions. Primary projection regions in the sensory system are the first cortical area to receive and process sensory information. The primary motor cortex contains the cell bodies of upper motor neurons. Primary regions project to secondary regions, which then project to tertiary regions. As information moves from primary to secondary and on to tertiary regions, it becomes elaborated and more highly processed. For example, the primary visual cortex sees individual stimuli in the environment. The secondary visual cortex connects adjacent stimuli to see a line and the tertiary visual cortex puts sequential lines together to form the perception that an object is moving in the visual field. Similarly, the supplementary (tertiary) motor cortex selects a movement goal, the premotor (secondary) cortex formulates a strategy for achieving that goal, and the primary motor cortex activates the upper motor neurons necessary to produce the desired muscular contractions.

The primary functions controlled from within the frontal lobe include movement, memory, emotion, and intellect. The frontal lobe contains the primary motor area (precentral gyrus, area 4 of Brodmann), as well as premotor and supplementary motor areas (6, 8); Broca's area (inferior frontal gyrus, 44, 45), which controls speech production; and prefrontal association areas (9, 10, 11). The primary function controlled from within the parietal lobe is sensation. The parietal lobe contains the primary sensory cortex (postcentral gyrus, 1, 2, 3), and secondary and tertiary sensory areas (5, 7). The primary function controlled from within the occipital lobe is vision and it contains the primary visual cortex (banks of the calcarine sulcus, 17) and visual association areas (18, 19). The primary functions controlled from within the temporal lobe are speech comprehension, hearing, and memory, and it contains Wernicke's area (the posterior portion of area 22) and the primary auditory cortex (Heschl's gyri, 41, 42). The primary cortical projection region for the limbic system is the cingulate gyrus (24, 33) on the medial aspect of the hemisphere. The parietal, temporal, and occipital lobes also contain association areas (19, 21, 22, 37, 39, 40). Association areas constitute by far the largest area of the cerebral cortex and their function is to integrate information from multiple systems to form abstract perceptions.

The Ventricular System

The ventricular system is the remnant of the hollow neural tube from which the central nervous system developed. All six regions of the central nervous system contain elements of the ventricular system. The lateral ventricles are located in the cerebral hemispheres. The third ventricle is located in the diencephalon. The cerebral aqueduct passes through the midbrain. The fourth ventricle separates the cerebellum from the pons and medulla and the central canal extends into the spinal cord. Chapter 21 contains a thorough discussion of the ventricular system.

a	Right hemisphere
b	Left hemisphere
c	Medial longitudinal fissure
d	Corpus callosum
e	Pons
f	Cerebellum
g	Medulla
h	Sulci
i	Gyri
j	Cerebral cortex
k	White matter (projection fibers)
l	Internal capsule
m	Lateral ventricle
n	Third ventricle
p	Insular cortex
q	Lateral fissure
r	Claustrum
s	Thalamus
t	Amygdala
u	Hypothalamus
v	Hippocampus
w	*Basal ganglia*
w^1	Caudate nucleus
w^2	Putamen
w^3	Globus pallidus

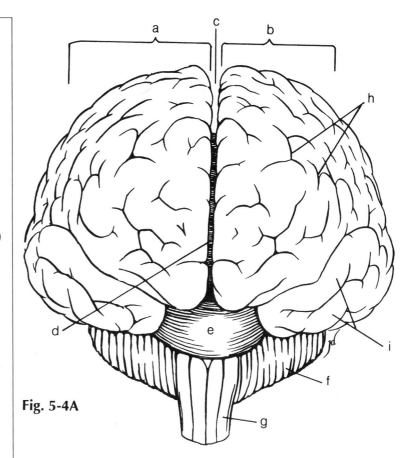

Fig. 5-4A

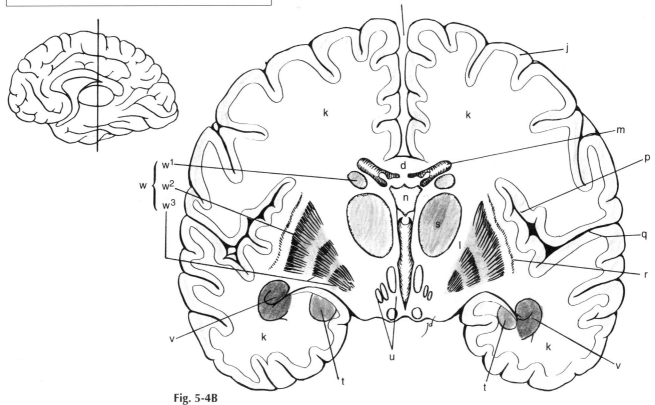

Fig. 5-4B

43

Protective Coverings

The central nervous system is the most highly protected organ in the human body. It is encased in a hard protective shell (the cranium and vertebral column); sealed in a tough, three-layer fibrous covering (the meninges); and suspended inside a hydraulic cylinder (the cerebrospinal fluid), all of which is designed to protect it from external trauma. Neurons in the central nervous system have the consistency of firm oatmeal. Thus, the brain gets its shape from the vessel within which it is housed. If the cranium were triangular, the brain would be triangular.

The meninges consist of a flexible, three-layered membrane (pia mater, arachnoid, dura mater; Fig. 5-5) that envelops the entire central nervous system. The pia mater is a transparently thin layer of connective tissue intimately attached to the surface of the brain and spinal cord, dipping into every sulcus and fissure. It is a vascular layer that contains blood vessels whose branches nourish the superficial tissue.

The arachnoid is a thin, avascular, honeycomb membrane between the pia and dura. The subarachnoid space contains cerebrospinal fluid and large blood vessels. In several locations the subarachnoid space is enlarged to form cisterns. The cisterna magna is located dorsal to the medulla and inferior to the cerebellum.

The pontine and interpeduncular cisterns are located in the anterior brain stem, and the superior cistern is located posterior to the midbrain. The spinal (lumbar) cistern is located caudal to the spinal cord between the second lumbar and second sacral vertebral levels and contains the cauda equina.

The dura mater is the superficial layer of the meninges. It consists of tough, nonelastic collagen fibers. The outer surface of the dura is continuous with the periosteum of the cranium, and the inner surface forms two sheets that penetrate deep within each hemisphere. The falx cerebri extends to the bottom of the medial longitudinal fissure and separates left and right hemispheres. The tentorium cerebelli penetrates to the dorsal surface of the midbrain and separates the cerebellum from the occipital lobes. The dura mater reattaches to the foramen magnum and then descends to envelop the spinal cord. It also encases each pair of spinal nerves as they exit the vertebral column. Unlike neural tissue, the dura mater is innervated with pain receptors and it has been implicated in some cases of low back and head pain.

The filum terminale is an extension of the meninges that anchors the caudal end of the spinal cord within the central canal. It extends from the conus medullaris to the dorsal surface of the second sacral vertebra.

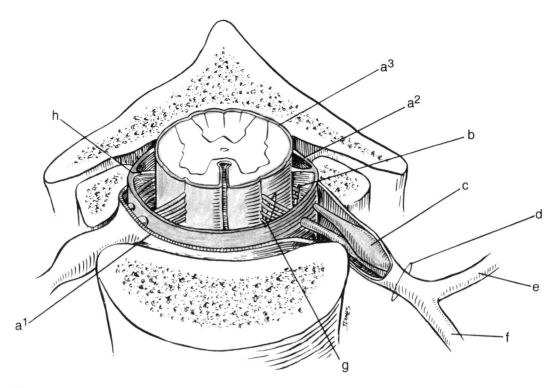

Fig. 5-5

a	*Meninges*
a¹	Dura mater
a²	Arachnoid
a³	Pia mater
b	Dorsal roots
c	Dorsal root ganglia
d	Spinal nerve
e	Dorsal ramus
f	Ventral ramus
g	Ventral roots
h	Denticulate ligament

6 The Peripheral Nervous System

Overview

The peripheral nervous system includes all neuromuscular and neuroendocrine structures lying outside the cranium and vertebral column (cranial and spinal nerves as well as sensory receptors). Peripheral structures extend the functional capacity of the nervous system. Sensory receptors respond to energy changes in the environment, perform preliminary analysis, and provide the central nervous system with the information necessary to formulate a perception of what is happening in the immediate environment both inside and outside the body. This information is used to formulate adaptive responses that work toward the accomplishment of a preselected goal. These responses are executed by effector organs (muscles and glands), which are at the command of the central nervous system via efferent neurons in peripheral nerves.

Functional Components of Peripheral Nerves

The peripheral nervous system conveys sensory and motor information to and from structures of the body wall and limbs as well as the hollow organs of the body. Afferent and efferent neurons to skeletal muscles, skin, bones, and joints are referred to collectively as the somatic nervous system while those to and from the hollow organs are referred to as the visceral nervous system. As a rule, peripheral nerves contain all four types of fibers (somatic sensory, somatic motor, visceral sensory, and visceral motor).

General afferent fibers are sensory neurons with their cell body located in the dorsal root ganglion (first-order neurons). Cell bodies are round and contain a single process that splits into distal and proximal axons (pseudomonopolar cells). The distal axon travels in a peripheral nerve to innervate a sensory organ and the proximal axon enters the central nervous system via the dorsal root. General somatic afferent (GSA) fibers convey information about pain, temperature, and touch from receptors located in the skin as well as proprioceptive information from receptors found in muscles, tendons, and joints (exteroceptive information). General visceral afferent (GVA) fibers convey sensory information from the hollow organs of the body (interoceptive information). General efferent fibers are motor neurons with their cell body located in the spinal cord or autonomic ganglia. General somatic efferent (GSE) fibers convey motor commands to striated skeletal muscles. The cell bodies of alpha, beta, and gamma motor neurons are located in lamina IX of the ventral horn; axons exit the spinal cord via the ventral roots and travel in peripheral nerves to innervate muscle fibers. General visceral efferent (GVE) fibers consist of the preganglionic and postganglionic autonomic fibers that innervate smooth muscle and cardiac muscle and regulate glandular secretion. The cell bodies of preganglionic sympathetic fibers are located in lamina VII, which forms the lateral horn, extending from T1 to L2 and cranial nerves III, VII, IX, and X. The cell bodies of preganglionic parasympathetic fibers are located in a similar region of the spinal cord between S2 and S4 as well as the brain stem. The axons of preganglionic autonomic fibers, both sympathetic and parasympathetic, synapse with the cell body of postganglionic fibers located in paravertebral and prevertebral ganglia.

Table 6-1 Classification of Nerve Fibers

Fibers	Diameter (μ)	Conduction Velocity, m/s	Role/Receptors Innervated
		Sensory	
Ia (A-alpha)	12–20	70–120	Primary afferents of muscle spindle
Ib (A-alpha)	12–20	70–120	Golgi tendon organs
II (A-beta)	5–14	30–70	Secondary afferents of muscle spindle
			Touch, pressure, and vibratory receptors
III (A-delta)	2–7	12–30	Touch and pressure receptors
			Pain and temperature receptors
IV (C)	0.5–1.0	0.5–2.0	Pain and temperature receptors
			Unmyelinated fibers
		Motor	
Alpha (A-alpha)	12–20	15–120	Alpha motor neurons
Gamma (A-gamma)	2–10	10–45	Gamma motor neurons
Preganglionic autonomic (B)	>3	3–15	Thinly myelinated preganglionic autonomic fibers
Postganglionic autonomic (C)	1	2	Unmyelinated postganglionic autonomic fibers

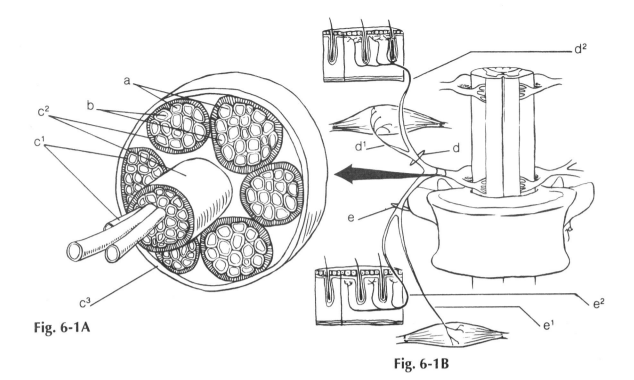

Fig. 6-1A

Fig. 6-1B

a	Sensory fiber
b	Motor fiber
c	*Neural coverings*
c^1	Endoneurium
c^2	Perineurium
c^3	Epineurium
d	Dorsal ramus
d^1	Muscular branch
d^2	Cutaneous branch
e	Ventral ramus
e^1	Muscular branch
e^2	Cutaneous branch
f	*Brachial plexus*
g	Upper trunk
h	Lateral division
i	Musculocutaneous nerve
j	Median nerve
k	Middle trunk
l	Posterior division
m	Axillary nerve
n	Radial nerve
p	Lower trunk
q	Anterior and medial divisions
r	Ulnar nerve

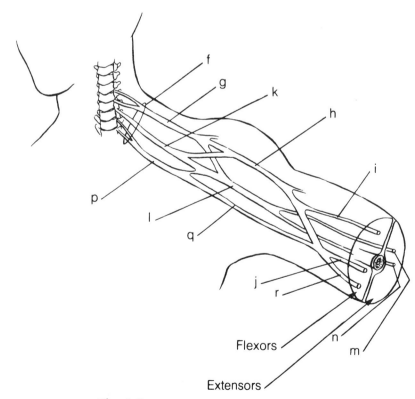

Flexors

Extensors

Fig. 6-2

Classification of Nerve Fibers

Nerve fibers can be classified according to fiber diameter, thickness of the myelin sheath, and conduction velocity. Generally, the larger the diameter of the fiber and the thicker the myelin sheath, the faster the conduction velocity. Currently, two systems are used to classify nerve fibers (Table 6-1). The first system uses conduction velocity to divide fibers into three groups: A, B, and C. A and B fibers are myelinated while C fibers are unmyelinated. On the basis of conduction velocity, A fibers are subdivided into alpha, beta, gamma, and delta classes. Alpha fibers innervate extrafusal muscle fibers, beta fibers innervate both extrafusal and intrafusal muscle fibers, gamma fibers innervate intrafusal muscle fibers, and delta fibers innervate sensory receptors of touch, pressure, pain, and temperature. Extrafusal muscle is striated muscle located outside the muscle spindle and intrafusal muscle is striated muscle located inside the muscle spindle. B fibers are small-diameter, thinly myelinated, preganglionic, autonomic motor fibers. C fibers are subdivided into two classes: sC (postganglionic efferent sympathetic C fibers) and drC (afferent dorsal root C fibers).

The second classification system deals only with sensory fibers and is subdivided into four groups (I, II, III, IV) on the basis of fiber diameter and site of origin. Group I fibers are subdivided into Ia, which originate from muscle spindles, and Ib, which originate from Golgi tendon organs. Group II fibers transmit impulses from encapsulated skin and joint receptors monitoring touch, pressure, and temperature as well as secondary endings from muscle spindles. Groups III and IV contain nonmyelinated fibers that transmit impulses from nonencapsulated endings monitoring pain, touch, and pressure.

Structure of Peripheral Nerves

The peripheral nervous system, like the central nervous system, is made up of neural tissue (nerve cells and their processes) and nonneural tissue (neuroglia and blood vessels). Peripheral nerves consist of mixed sensory and motor fibers that extend from spinal nerves to effector organs (Fig. 6-1A). Individual axons, including their myelin or neurilemma, are sheathed in the delicate endoneurium. Groups of axons are organized into bundles by the perineurium. The epineurium binds the bundles together and provides a protective covering for the entire nerve. These three layers of fibrous coverings provide support for both neural and nonneural tissue, provide the tensile strength of the nerve, and attach peripheral nerves to surrounding fascia.

Once outside the vertebral column, the spinal nerve bifurcates into dorsal and ventral rami (Fig. 6-1B). The pattern of distribution of these rami is fairly common among segmental levels with each ramus having smaller muscular and cutaneous branches. Muscular branches supply the four types of fibers to muscles and joints while cutaneous branches supply them to the overlying skin. The dorsal ramus supplies sensory and motor fibers to the deep musculature of the back, overlying skin, and fascia; the ventral ramus provides sensory and motor fibers to the rest of the body. This simple dorsal and ventral division is adequate for the trunk but becomes more complex at the extremities.

Table 6-2   Distribution of Peripheral Nerves

Nerve	General Function
Upper extremity	
Musculocutaneous	Sensory: dorsal and ventral surfaces of the radial half of the forearm
	Motor: elbow and shoulder flexion
Axillary	Sensory: distal two thirds of the posterior aspect of deltoid and adjacent long head of the triceps brachii
	Motor: shoulder abduction and external rotation
Median	Sensory: palmar surface of thumb and first three fingers
	Motor: finger and wrist flexion
Ulnar	Sensory: fourth and fifth fingers
	Motor: intrinsic hand muscles
Radial	Sensory: dorsum of the hand
	Motor: forearm, wrist, and hand extension
Lower extremity	
Femoral	Sensory: anterior aspect of thigh and medial aspect of leg
	Motor: hip flexion and knee extension
Obturator	Sensory: usually nonexistent
	Motor: hip adduction
Sciatic	Sensory: posterior aspect of thigh and portion of leg below the knee
	Motor: knee flexion and all ankle and foot motion
Tibial	Sensory: posterior part of leg and sole of foot
	Motor: foot extension and toe flexion
Peroneal	Sensory: lateral aspect of leg and dorsum of foot
	Motor: foot flexion and toe extension

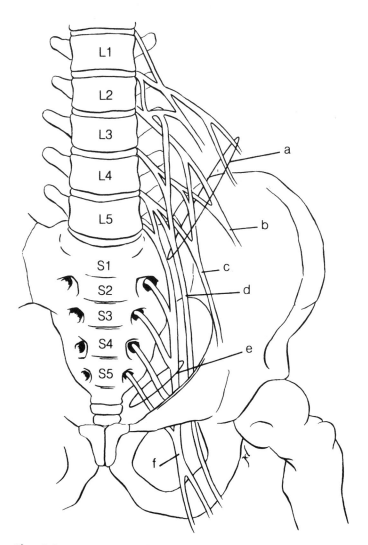

Fig. 6-3

a	*Lumbar plexus*
b	Lateral femoral cutaneous
c	Femoral nerve
d	Obturator nerve
e	*Sacral plexus*
f	Sciatic nerve
g	Tibial nerve
h	Medial plantar nerve
i	Lateral plantar nerve
j	Common peroneal nerve
k	Superficial peroneal nerve
l	Deep peroneal nerve

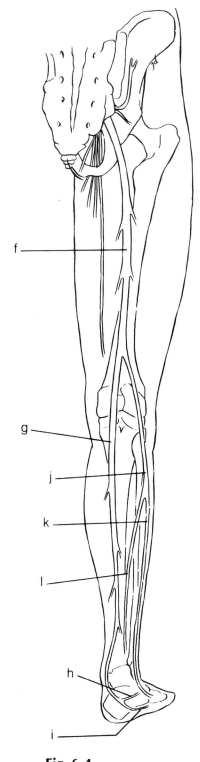

Fig. 6-4

The nerves that supply the musculoskeletal structures of the upper extremity are derived from a neural network called the brachial plexus (Fig. 6-2), which is located deep beneath the clavicle and extends through the apex of the axilla. The brachial plexus consists of the ventral rami of the fifth through eighth cervical and first thoracic spinal nerves (C5–T1). In the axilla three primary nerve trunks and four divisions are formed. The upper trunk supplies the lateral division, which innervates flexor muscles via the musculocutaneous and median nerves; the middle trunk supplies the posterior division, which innervates extensor muscles via the axillary and radial nerves; and the lower trunk supplies the anterior or medial division, which innervates flexor muscles via the ulnar and median nerves.

The nerves that supply the musculoskeletal structures of the lower extremity are derived from two neural networks, called the lumbar and sacral plexuses (Fig. 6-3). The lumbar plexus is located among fibers of the psoas muscle in the posterior abdominal wall and derived from the ventral rami of the first through fourth lumbar spinal nerves. (L1–L4). The lumbar plexus innervates the lower abdominal wall, genitalia, and thigh. The principal nerves of this plexus are the lateral femoral cutaneous nerve, which innervates the lateral thigh from hip to knee; the obturator nerve, which innervates the adductor muscles of the thigh and overlying skin; and the femoral nerve, which innervates the flexors of the hip, extensors of the knee, and cutaneous branches of the medial thigh. The larger sacral plexus is located in the posterolateral pelvic wall and passes to the leg through the obturator foramen. The fourth and fifth lumbar and first through third sacral spinal nerves form the sacral plexus (L4–S3), which innervates the perineum, pelvis, posterior thigh, leg, and foot. The principal nerve of the sacral plexus is the sciatic nerve (largest peripheral nerve in the body), which innervates the hamstring muscles and then, just above the knee, divides into the tibial and common peroneal nerves (Fig. 6-4). The tibial nerve innervates the gastrocnemius and soleus muscles, then crosses under the foot and divides into the medial and lateral plantar nerves, which innervates toe muscles. The common peroneal nerve divides into a superficial branch, which innervates the peroneal muscles, and a deep branch, which innervates the tibialis anterior and long toe extensors.

Table 6-2 describes the distribution of major peripheral nerves.

Patterns of Cutaneous Innervation

Sensory information is conveyed to the central nervous system via afferent fibers of cutaneous nerves that enter the spinal cord in the dorsal roots or the brain stem in the sensory component of cranial nerves. The afferent fibers of individual spinal nerves transmit sensory information from a restricted body region, called a dermatome (Fig. 6-5). Although individual dermatomes have definite boundaries, adjacent dermatomes overlap so that any given skin area, except the back of the head, is innervated by more than one spinal or cranial nerve, usually three and sometimes four. Thus, damage to a single dorsal root or cranial nerve will not result in complete abolition of sensation (anesthesia) in any region of the body. Sensory loss (hypoesthesia) may result from damage to the dorsal roots of adjacent spinal nerves or the sensory component of cranial nerves. The overlapping of adjacent dermatomes differs for individual sensory modalities. Overlap is greater for touch than for pain or thermal senses. A composite map of touch dermatomes and their overlap provides an overview of the cutaneous innervation pattern.

Clinical Aspects

The symptoms produced by lesions of peripheral and spinal nerves differ in the completeness and distribution of symptoms. Because peripheral nerves are formed distal to a plexus, transection will result in the loss of all motor and autonomic function supplied by that nerve. Sensation may only be diminished because of overlapping innervation from adjacent dermatomes. The distribution of deficits will be myotomal or dermatomal. Because cervical and lumbar spinal nerves feed into a plexus, and contribute fibers to more than one peripheral nerve, lesion of a spinal nerve produces only weakness with diminished sensation and autonomic function. However, these symptoms are more widespread than those of a peripheral nerve lesion. For example, transection of the axillary nerve completely paralyzes the deltoid and teres minor muscles and destroys their autonomic innervation whereas lesion of the C5 spinal nerve decreases the strength of all muscles innervated by the phrenic, long thoracic, dorsal scapular, subscapular, suprascapular, thoracodorsal, lateral and medial pectoral, axillary, musculocutaneous, radical, and median nerves. Because these nerves also contain fibers from other segmental levels, the strength of the muscles they innervate is only decreased, not abolished. Approximately 50 percent of the motor fibers in the axillary nerve originate from C6; thus, following a lesion of the C5 spinal nerve, clinical assessment of the strength of the deltoid and teres minor muscles would be approximately fair. The distribution of sensory deficits following the two lesions would also differ. Both lesions would produce sensory deficits in the respective dermatomes; however, the C5 dermatome is roughly four times larger than the axillary dermatome.

The motor and sensory deficits following lesion of the brachial plexus vary considerably, depending on the location of the lesion and its extent. Following injury to the trunks, the symptoms occur in a segmental distribution and two syndromes are recognized. Upper trunk syndrome involves the muscles innervated by C5 and C6, namely the deltoid, biceps, brachialis, brachioradialis, supinator, teres major, teres minor,

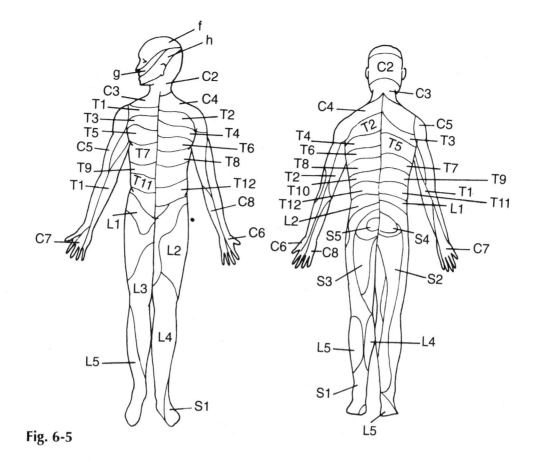

Fig. 6-5

(f–h)	Dermatomes of face, trigeminal nerve (CNV)
f	Ophthalmic
g	Maxillary
h	Mandibular

supraspinatus, and infraspinatus. Because of the muscles involved, an individual has difficulty in elevating and externally rotating the arm and extreme difficulty in flexing and supinating the forearm. Because of overlapping sensory innervation, sensory deficits are usually limited to the deltoid region and lateral aspect of the arm. Lower trunk syndrome is relatively rare and primarily affects the intrinsic muscles of the hand innervated by C8 and T1. The palmaris longus and long finger flexors are usually involved, producing functional deficits involving finger and wrist movements. The sensory loss is along the medial aspect of the arm, forearm, and hand. If the preganglionic sympathetic fibers of T1 are involved in the injury, there may be drooping of the eyelid and narrowing of the space between upper and lower eyelids (palpebral fissure) and constriction of the pupil (Horner's syndrome).

Lesion of the cords of the brachial plexus produces symptoms similar to those of peripheral nerve injuries, except that they are multiple and often incomplete. Thus, a lesion of the posterior cord involves the radial and axillary, and often the thoracodorsal and subscapular nerves. Lesion of the lateral cord involves the musculocutaneous and lateral portion of the median nerve. Lesion of the medial cord involves the ulnar nerve and medial portion of the median nerve, as well as the medial brachial and antebrachial cutaneous nerves.

The causes and grades of peripheral nerve injury as well as the recovery of function are discussed in the clinical aspects section of Chap. 2, The Neuron.

7 Cranial Nerves

Overview

Cranial nerves are functionally analogous to spinal nerves; that is, the 12 pairs of cranial nerves are the peripheral nerves of the brain and serve the somatic, visceral, and autonomic needs of the face, head, neck, and select abdominal viscera. All but two cranial nerves (olfactory and optic) connect to the brain stem. Some cranial nerves contain only sensory fibers, others only motor fibers, and some contain both sensory and motor fibers. Sensory fibers have their cell bodies located in peripheral ganglia with proximal axons that enter the brain stem and synapse in sensory nuclei and distal axons that innervate receptors. Motor fibers are lower motor neurons with their cell bodies located in the motor nucleus of the corresponding cranial nerve. The sensory ganglia of cranial nerves and the dorsal root ganglia of spinal nerves both develop from the neural crest during embryonic development. Likewise, the motor nuclei of cranial nerves and the ventral horn of the spinal cord both develop from the basal plate in the neural tube.

Classification of Cranial Nerves

Many of the cranial nerves can be classified into the same functional categories as spinal nerves. Four of the

Table 7-1   Cranial Nerve Functional Components and Clinical Tests

Nerve	Number	Components	Major Functions	Clinical Tests
Olfactory	I	Special visceral afferent	Smell	Odor categories, test ipsilaterally
Optic	II	Special somatic afferent	Vision	Visual acuity, test ipsilaterally
Oculomotor	III	General somatic efferent	Movements of the eyes	Cardinal planes of gaze
		General visceral efferent (parasympathetic)	Pupillary constriction and accommodation	Pupillary reactivity
Trochlear	IV	General somatic efferent	Movements of the eyes	Cardinal planes of gaze
Trigeminal	V	Special visceral efferent	Muscles of mastication and eardrum tension	Motor: open and close jaw against resistance Sensory: facial sensation, corneal reflex
		General somatic efferent	General sensations from anterior half of head, including face, nose, mouth, and meninges	
Abducens	VI	General somatic efferent	Movements of the eyes	Cardinal planes of gaze
Facial	VII	Special visceral efferent	Muscles of facial expression and tension of ossicles	Smile Wrinkle brow
		General visceral efferent (parasympathetic)	Lacrimation and salivation	
		Special visceral afferent	Taste	
		General visceral afferent	Visceral sensory	
Vestibulocochlear	VIII	Special somatic afferent	Hearing and equilibrium reception	Vestibular: caloric, postrotary nystagmus Cochlear: Weber, audiometric, evoked potential
Glossopharyngeal	IX	Special visceral efferent	Swallowing movements and laryngeal control	"Say ah" Gag reflex, test ipsilaterally
		General visceral efferent (parasympathetic)	Salivation	
		Special visceral afferent	Taste	
		General visceral afferent	Visceral sensory	
Vagus nerve and cranial root of XI	X	General visceral efferent (parasympathetic)	Parasympathetics to thoracic and abdominal viscera	Cough
		Special visceral afferent	Taste	
		General visceral afferent	Visceral sensory	
Spinal accessory (spinal root)	XI	Special visceral efferent	Movements of shoulder and head	Shoulder shrug Resisted head rotation
Hypoglossal	XII	General somatic efferent	Movements of tongue	Stick tongue out and move side to side

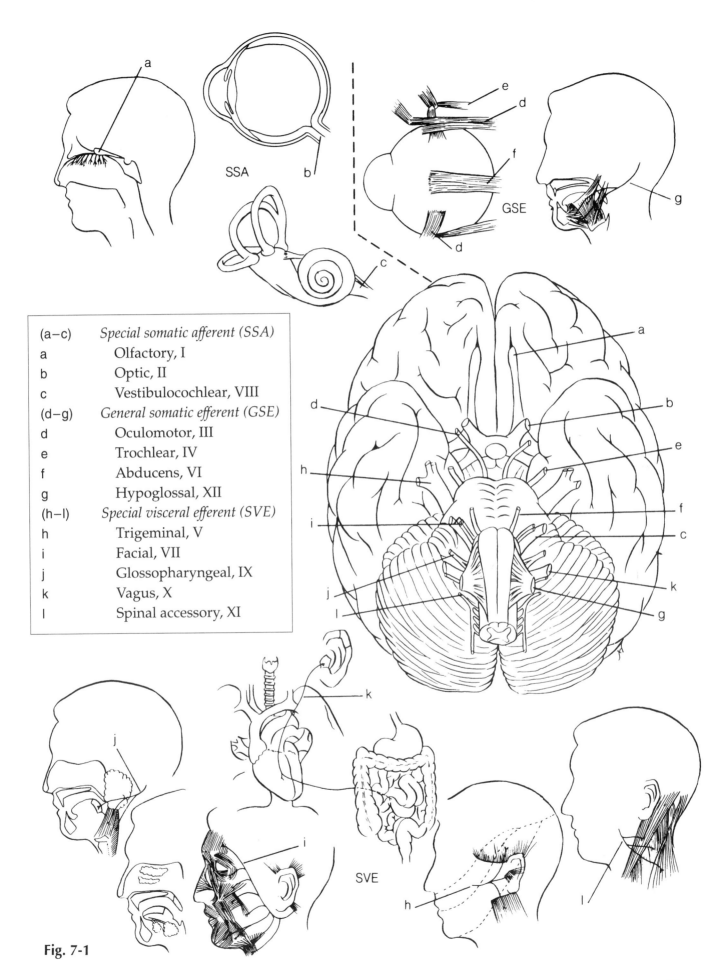

SSA

GSE

(a–c)	*Special somatic afferent (SSA)*
a	Olfactory, I
b	Optic, II
c	Vestibulocochlear, VIII
(d–g)	*General somatic efferent (GSE)*
d	Oculomotor, III
e	Trochlear, IV
f	Abducens, VI
g	Hypoglossal, XII
(h–l)	*Special visceral efferent (SVE)*
h	Trigeminal, V
i	Facial, VII
j	Glossopharyngeal, IX
k	Vagus, X
l	Spinal accessory, XI

SVE

Fig. 7-1

53

categories are shared by both types of nerves and three are specialized to cranial nerves. The four shared categories, derived from the embryonic neural tube, are the general somatic afferent (GSA), which carries sensory information from the musculoskeletal system; general somatic efferent (GSE), which carries motor commands to musculoskeletal structures; general visceral afferent (GVA), which carries sensory information from visceral organs (circulatory system, muscle spindles, tendon organs); and general visceral efferent (GVE), which carries commands to the visceral organs (involuntary muscles and glands). The categories specialized to cranial nerves are the special somatic afferent (SSA), which functions in vision, audition, and equilibrium; special visceral afferent (SVA), which functions in olfaction (smell) and gustation (taste); and special visceral efferent (SVE, branchial), which innervates voluntary muscles of the head and neck. Although most cranial nerves contain both general and special functions, spinal nerves contain only general functions.

Even though cranial nerves are numbered I through XII from rostral to caudal (Fig. 7-1), they can be classified according to their functional components and are usually tested according to these categories. Table 7-1 lists the cranial nerves with their functional components and their clinical tests. Figure 7-2 shows the location of the sensory nuclei of the cranial nerves and Fig. 7-3 shows the location of the motor nuclei of the cranial nerves.

Special Afferent Nerves

The special afferent nerves serve the special senses: smell, sight, taste, hearing, and balance (equilibrium). This class of special afferents contains two subgroups: SVA and SSA.

Special Visceral Afferent Nerves

The olfactory nerve (I) is the only special visceral afferent nerve. It is composed of the axons of bipolar olfactory receptor cells. Bipolar cells are first-order neurons that act as receptor and transducer for chemical stimuli. Each olfactory neuron has a life cycle of approximately 30 days after which it is replaced by maturing basal cells in the olfactory mucosa. Basal cells are continuously differentiating into new neurons that form new synaptic connections in the olfactory bulb. The central pathway for olfaction includes an olfactory bulb and stalk located on the ventral surface of the frontal lobe that projects directly to the amygdala and olfactory cortex (area 28) without passing through the thalamus. Beyond sensing and perceiving odors, the olfactory has strong projections to other regions of the brain (rhinencephalon) and has strong reflex connections capable of producing salivation, secretion of digestive enzymes, or vomiting. Chap. 16 contains a complete discussion of the olfactory system.

Clinical Aspects The olfactory nerve is tested clinically by unilateral presentation of an olfactory stimulus (odorant) to test for perception. Lesions, should they occur, are on the side of deficit.

The olfactory system is of limited clinical importance in humans, although two types of pathology do occur: loss of smell and olfactory hallucinations. Loss of smell (anosmia) may result from infections (including the common cold), trauma, neoplasms, metabolic disorders, and drug ingestion. Diminished sensitivity, if bilaterally symmetrical, is of little clinical importance; however, bilateral imbalance can help to establish the laterality of neurological problems to the side of the diminished sensitivity. Because olfactory and gustatory systems work together, complete anosmia results in an inability to recognize flavors. In addition, the sense of smell may diminish in the later decades of life because the threshold to detect various odors is considerably higher in older people. Finally, skull fractures involving the cribriform plate may tear the olfactory stalk. If anterior-posterior shear force is great enough, olfactory fibers from both hemispheres may be involved. Such fractures may permit cerebrospinal fluid to leak through the nose and infectious agents to enter the central nervous system.

Special Somatic Afferent Nerves

Special somatic afferent nerves include the optic and vestibulocochlear nerves.

The Optic Nerve (II) The optic nerve consists of axons of ganglion cells from the retina and is actually a tract of the central nervous system. Fibers from the nasal half of each retina cross the midline in the optic chiasm and project to the thalamus as the optic tract. A complete discussion of the optic nerve can be found in Chap. 12, Visual System.

Clinical Aspects Clinical tests of the optic nerve are tests of visual acuity, often performed with a Snellen chart.

Because the optic nerve is actually a tract of the central nervous system, myelinated by oligodendrocytes, it is susceptible to demyelinating disease (multiple sclerosis). Cerebrovascular accidents regularly involve the optic tract as it passes the junction of the internal carotid and middle cerebral arteries. The extent and precise location of damage to the optic tract will determine the resulting visual deficit. Tumors of the central nervous system may also affect the optic nerve. If the entire optic nerve is sectioned, all vision originating from that eye is lost (ipsilateral monocular blindness). The most common lesion of the optic chiasm involves the crossing fibers from the nasal portion of the retina, which produce a loss of both temporal visual fields (bitemporal hemianopia). Rarely, the uncrossing fibers from the temporal portions of the retina will be damaged in the chiasm, producing a loss of both nasal visual fields (binasal hemianopia). Lesions of the optic tract, lateral geniculate body, or optic radiations on one side produce homonymous defects in the opposite visual field: right or left homonymous hemianopia. See Chap. 12 for a complete discussion of clinical aspects of the visual system.

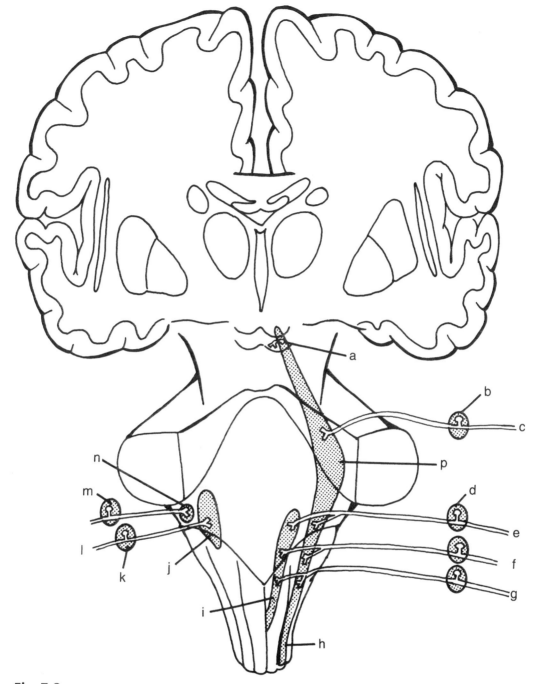

Fig. 7-2

a	Mesencephalic nucleus of V	i	Solitary tract and nucleus
b	Trigeminal ganglion	j	Vestibular nuclei
c	Trigeminal nerve (V)	k	Vestibular ganglion
d	Geniculate ganglion	l	Vestibulocochlear nerve
e	Facial nerve	m	Spiral ganglion
f	Glossopharyngeal nerve	n	Cochlear nuclei
g	Vagus nerve	p	Principal sensory nucleus of V
h	Spinal tract and nucleus of V		

The Vestibulocochlear Nerve (VIII) The vestibulocochlear nerve functions as two separate nerves. The vestibular portion transmits proprioceptive information concerned with equilibrium and the orientation of the head in space. It consists of bipolar neurons with their cell bodies located in the vestibular ganglion. Peripheral processes receive their input from hair cells in the crista (in ampullae of the semicircular ducts) and in the maculae (of the utricle and saccule). Central processes terminate in the four vestibular nuclei in the ipsilateral medulla and pons. The cochlear portion transmits information about exteroceptive stimuli concerned with hearing. It consists of bipolar neurons with their cell bodies located in the spiral ganglion. Peripheral processes receive their input from hair cells in the organ of Corti. Central processes terminate in the dorsal and central cochlear nuclei. A complete discussion of both portions of the nerve can be found in Chap. 14, Vestibular System, and Chap. 13, Auditory System.

Clinical Aspects Tests of the vestibular portion of the nerve are performed with caloric or thermal, oculocephalic reflexes (doll's eyes) and postrotary nystagmus tests. Tests of the cochlear portion of the nerve are performed by specialists using audiometric instruments and auditory evoked potentials.

Damage to the vestibular portion of the nerve produces disequilibrium, vertigo, and nystagmus. Nausea and vomiting may accompany these symptoms because of the connections between the vestibular and vagus nerves. The most common cause of damage to this nerve is produced by a tumor of the Schwann cells myelinating it (acoustic neuroma), which tends to also affect the cochlear component as well as the facial nerve. Damage to the cochlear component of the nerve produces ringing in the ears (tinnitus) followed by eventual ipsilateral deafness. Damage to the facial nerve produces weakness or paralysis of the muscles of facial expression, loss of taste from the anterior two thirds of the tongue, and a lack of stimulation of the salivary, mucosal, and lacrimal glands on the same side as the tumor. For a complete discussion of the clinical aspects of the vestibular system, see Chap. 14, and of the auditory system, see Chap. 13.

General Somatic Efferent Nerves

General somatic efferent nerves are motor nerves that innervate the voluntary muscles of the eye and eyelid (oculomotor, trochlear, and abducens) and tongue (hypoglossal). In addition to its GSE fibers, the oculomotor nerve contains parasympathetic (GVE) fibers to the ciliary and pupillary constrictor muscles.

Oculomotor (III), Trochlear (IV), and Abducens (VI) Nerves

Together, these cranial nerves control voluntary movement of the eyes. The central pathways for these nerves are linked in such a way that their simultaneous actions produce conjugate movements of the eyes (simultaneous movement of both eyes in the same direction). Lateral movement of the eyes, as used in tracking a moving car, requires simultaneous contraction of the lateral rectus from one eye and the medial rectus of the other. Each nerve also has proprioceptive (GSA) fibers, which have their cell bodies along the nerve, in the trigeminal ganglion, or in the mesencephalic nucleus of the trigeminal nerve. The oculomotor nerve also has preganglionic parasympathetic (GVE) fibers that synapse with postganglionic fibers in the ciliary ganglion. These fibers participate in the accommodation reflex that constricts the pupil in response to light. A complete discussion of the extraocular muscles can be found in Chap. 12, Visual System.

Hypoglossal Nerve (XII)

Lower motor neurons in the hypoglossal nerve have their cell bodies located in the hypoglossal nucleus in the brain stem and innervate the muscles of the ipsilateral tongue (genioglossus, styloglossus, and hypoglossus). The nerve also contains proprioceptive fibers from the lingual musculature (GSA), thought to arise from scattered neurons that have been found along the nerve.

Clinical Aspects The oculomotor, trochlear, and abducens nerves are tested together using the cardinal planes of gaze (horizontal, vertical, and diagonal). The hypoglossal nerve is tested by asking the client to stick the tongue straight out and then move it from side to side.

A complete lesion of the oculomotor nerve produces the following: double vision (diplopia), drooping and inability to lift the eyelid (ptosis), dilated pupil (mydriasis) with lack of the accommodation reflex, pupils of unequal size (anisocoria), abduction of the ipsilateral eye, and inability to move inward, upward, or downward (external strabismus). A complete lesion of the trochlear nerve produces the following: vertical diplopia, head tilt to the side opposite the paralyzed muscle to accommodate the diplopia, and limitation of eye movement on looking down, which makes descending stairs very difficult. Because the trochlear nerve is crossed, symptoms are seen in the side opposite the lesion. A complete lesion of the abducens nerve produces the following: horizontal diplopia with adduction of the ipsilateral eye and inability to abduct the affected eye past the midline.

Lesion of the hypoglossal nerve produces an ipsilateral lower motor paralysis of the tongue. Early fibrillations are replaced by muscle atrophy and wrinkling on the side of the lesion. When protruded, the tongue deviates to the paralyzed side.

Special Visceral Nerves

The special visceral nerves (trigeminal, facial, glossopharyngeal, vagus, and spinal accessory) are mixed in function. The special visceral efferent (SVE) component

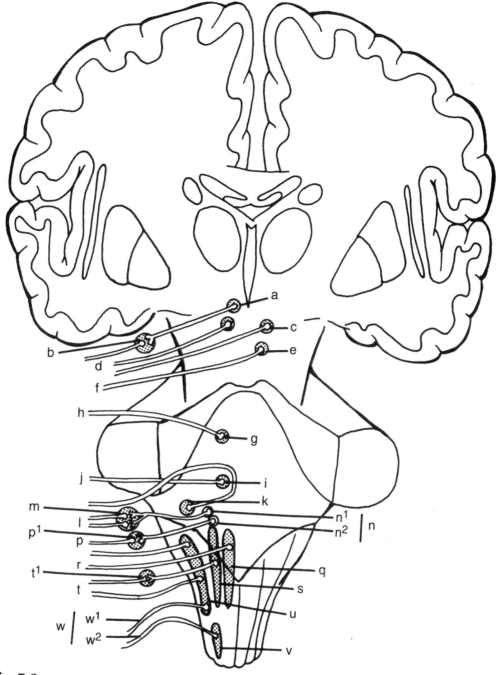

Fig. 7-3

a	Accessory oculomotor nucleus (Edinger-Westphal)	j	Abducens nerve (VI)	q	Hypoglossal nucleus
		k	Motor nucleus of VII	r	Hypoglossal nerve (XII)
		l	Facial nerve (VII)	s	Dorsal vagal nucleus
b	Ciliary ganglion	m	Pterygopalatine and submandibular ganglia	t	Vagus nerve (X)
c	Oculomotor nucleus			t¹	Terminal ganglia
d	Oculomotor nerve (III)	n	Salivatory nucleus	u	Nucleus ambiguus
e	Trochlear nucleus	n¹	Superior	v	Spinal nucleus of XI
f	Trochlear nerve (IV)	n²	Inferior	w	Accessory nerve
g	Motor nucleus of V	p	Glossopharyngeal nerve (IX)	w¹	Cranial root
h	Trigeminal nerve (V)			w²	Spinal root
i	Abducent nucleus	p¹	Otic ganglion		

of these nerves is referred to as visceral, not because the nerves are part of the autonomic system but because the actions they regulate, eating and breathing, are considered visceral functions. SVE fibers innervate the muscles of the branchiomeric arches of the face from the eyes to the chin. The facial, glossopharyngeal, and vagus nerves also contain SVA fibers subserving taste, parasympathetic fibers (GVE), and GVA fibers.

Trigeminal Nerve (V)

The trigeminal nerve (the largest cranial nerve) branches into three divisions: ophthalmic, maxillary, and mandibular. Unlike spinal dermatomes, there is no overlap in these adjacent dermatomes. Sensory fibers enter the brain stem at the level of the midpons as the sensory root and motor fibers exit at the adjacent motor root.

The sensory root carries two sources of information: exteroceptive and proprioceptive. Exteroceptive sensory afferents (GSA) are first-order neurons with cell bodies located in the trigeminal ganglion. Distal axons innervate receptors located in the skin of the face, scalp anterior to a coronal plane through the ears, orbit, mucous membrane of the nasal and oral cavities, nasal sinus, teeth, and most of the dura. Proximal axons terminate in the principal sensory nucleus and the spinal trigeminal nucleus. Proprioceptive afferents are first-order neurons with cell bodies in the mesencephalic nucleus of the trigeminal nerve. The mesencephalic nucleus also receives proprioceptive fibers from the extraocular muscles. Distal axons innervate the muscles of mastication and pressure receptors in the periodontal ligaments and teeth via the mandibular nerve. Proximal axons terminate in the motor nucleus of the trigeminal nerve. Some proprioceptive fibers establish monosynaptic connections with lower motor neurons in the motor nucleus of the trigeminal nerve to mediate the jaw-jerk reflex.

The motor root contains lower motor neurons with their cell bodies in the motor nucleus of the trigeminal nerve (SVE) that travel via the mandibular nerve and innervate the muscles of mastication (masseter, pterygoids, and temporalis), the tensor tympani, the tensor veli palatini, the mylohyoid, and the anterior belly of the digastric. These muscles arise embryologically from the first branchial arch.

Clinical Aspects The motor functions of the trigeminal nerve are tested by asking the client to open and close the jaw against resistance. The sensory functions of the nerve are tested with general sensory tests of the face, by dermatome, and by the corneal reflex (a contraction of the eyelids when the cornea is lightly touched).

A complete lesion of the trigeminal nerve produces the following symptoms: anesthesia and loss of general sensation in the three dermatomes of the face, which produces a loss of corneal reflex bilaterally; a lower motor neuron paralysis, which produces a loss of the jaw-jerk reflex; and relaxation of the ipsilateral muscles of facial expression, in which, on protrusion, the jaw will deviate toward the side of the lesion. Trigeminal neuralgia is sharp agonizing pain over the distribution of one or more of the branches of the trigeminal nerve. This condition, of unknown origin, may be accompanied by involuntary muscle contractions (tics) and disturbances of salivary secretion.

Facial Nerve (VII)

The facial nerve contains motor and sensory divisions. The motor division contains two types of fibers: SVE and GVE. Lower motor neurons with their cell bodies in the motor nucleus of the facial nerve (SVE) innervate the muscles of facial expression (orbicularis oculi, buccinator, stapedius, platysma, stylohyoid, and posterior belly of the digastric). These muscles originate from the second branchial arch. The parasympathetic preganglionic fibers (GVE) from the salivatory nucleus pass through the nervus intermedius and synapse with postganglionic neurons in the pterygopalatine and submandibular ganglia. Postganglionic neurons innervate lacrimal, oral, submaxillary, and sublingual glands as well as blood vessels.

The sensory division of the facial nerve contains two types of fibers: GSA and SVA. All first-order sensory neurons have their cell bodies located in the geniculate ganglion. The distal process of GSA fibers conveys information about pain and temperature from exteroceptors located in the external auditory meatus and skin of the ear. The central process of these fibers terminates in the nucleus of the spinal tract of the trigeminal nerve. The distal branch of SVA fibers innervates taste buds on the anterior two thirds of the tongue via the chorda tympani and lingual nerves. The central branch of these fibers passes through the nervus intermedius and terminates in the rostral portion of the nucleus solitarius.

Clinical Aspects The facial nerve is tested by asking the client to smile and wrinkle the brow. Bilateral asymmetry of smile is a positive test result.

Lesion of the facial nerve is seen primarily as lower motor neuron paralysis of the muscles of facial expression (Bell's palsy). Corneal sensitivity remains but the individual is unable to blink or close the eye. The eye requires protection from damage due to dehydration (eye patch). Lacrimation and salivation are impaired on the side of lesion. Taste is lost from the anterior two thirds of the tongue on the side of the lesion. Low tone sounds will be heard increasingly (hyperacusis) because the stapedius muscle that usually dampens them is paralyzed. The sensory component of the trigeminal nerve supplies the sensory limb of the corneal reflex and the facial nerve supplies the motor limb. Unilateral lesion of the facial nerve results in a contralateral blink response (consensual corneal reflex) when the involved eye is challenged. Parasympathetic involvement in a facial nerve lesion may produce increased lacrimal secretion in both eyes.

Lower motor neuron lesions (facial nerve) and upper

motor neuron lesions (corticobulbar and corticoreticular fibers) produce different effects on facial muscles. A lower motor neuron lesion paralyzes all the muscles of facial expression on the same side as the lesion. An upper motor neuron lesion paralyzes the facial muscles below the eye but not eyelid or forehead muscles on the side opposite the lesion.

Glossopharyngeal Nerve (IX)

The glossopharyngeal nerve contains fibers from five different functional categories. The cell bodies of GSA fibers are located in the superior ganglion of IX, with distal processes that innervate pain and temperature receptors in the external auditory meatus and skin over the ear. The proximal processes terminate in the nucleus of the spinal tract of the trigeminal nerve. The cell bodies of GVA fibers are located in the inferior (petrosal) ganglion, with distal processes that carry general sensory input (not taste) from the posterior third of the tongue and the pharynx. A special branch of these fibers innervates the carotid sinus (pressor receptors and arterial pressure receptors) and the carotid body (chemoreceptors, CO_2, and O_2 concentration in the blood). Most of the central processes terminate in the caudal part of the nucleus of the solitary tract. Other cell bodies in the inferior ganglion have peripheral processes that innervate taste buds on the posterior third of the tongue. Central processes of these SVA fibers terminate in the rostral portion of the nucleus of the solitary tract. SVE fibers with cell bodies in the nucleus ambiguus innervate the muscles that affect swallowing (pharyngeal and palatine muscles) and the muscle that elevates the upper pharynx (stylopharyngeus). This is the only skeletal muscle of the third branchial arch. Preganglionic parasympathetic (GVE) fibers from the inferior salivatory nucleus terminate in the otic ganglion. Postganglionic fibers innervate the parotid gland.

Clinical Aspects   The glossopharyngeal nerve is tested by asking the client to say "ah" and watching to see that the soft palate moves or by using a tongue blade to produce a gag reflex.

Lesion of the glossopharyngeal nerve produces the following symptoms: loss of sensation, including taste, from the posterior third of the tongue; loss of gag, palatal, uvular, and carotid reflexes; difficulty in swallowing (dysphagia); and deviation of the palate and uvula to the normal side.

Vagus Nerve (X)

The vagus contains fibers from five different functional categories. The cell bodies of GSA fibers are located in the superior (jugular) ganglion of X and distal processes conveying touch, pain, and temperature information from the skin of the auricle. The central processes of these neurons terminate in the spinal nucleus of V. The cell bodies of GVA fibers are located in the inferior (nodose) ganglion and distal processes convey general sensory information from the respiratory system (pharynx, larynx, trachea, and lungs), cardiovascular system (carotid body and sinus, heart, and various blood vessels), gastrointestinal tract, and dura mater in the posterior fossa. The proximal processes of these neurons terminate in the nucleus solitarius. The SVA fibers mediate taste. Their cell bodies are located in the inferior ganglion; distal processes innervate taste buds in the epiglottis via the internal laryngeal nerve. Central processes of these neurons also terminate in the nucleus solitarius. The GVE component consists of preganglionic parasympathetic fibers from the dorsal vagal nucleus that terminate on postganglionic neurons in the wall of the thoracic and abdominal viscera. Postganglionic fibers extend to cardiovascular, respiratory, and gastrointestinal organs, where they innervate glands, and cardiac and smooth muscle. The SVE output is by lower motor neurons from the nucleus ambiguus that innervate the voluntary muscles of the soft palate, pharynx, and intrinsic laryngeal muscles.

Clinical Aspects   The vagus nerve can be tested with the glossopharyngeal while producing a gag reflex or by asking the client to cough.

A complete unilateral lesion of the vagus nerve produces the following symptoms: flaccid soft palate, which produces a voice with a twang; difficulty in swallowing (dysphagia); a weak cough; and transient tachycardia. Bilateral lesions of the vagus nerve are usually fatal due to laryngeal paralysis.

Spinal Accessory Nerve (XI)

The accessory nerve contains two roots: bulbar (cranial) and spinal. Both roots contain SVE fibers. The cervical root has cell bodies located in the nucleus ambiguus and fibers accompanying the vagus nerve form the recurrent laryngeal nerve, which innervates the intrinsic laryngeal muscles. Fibers in the spinal root originate from anterior horn cells in segments C1 through C5 (spinal accessory nucleus). After exiting the spinal cord, fibers ascend on the lateral surface of the cord, pass rostrally through the foramen magnum, join with the cranial root in the jugular foramen, exit the skull with nerves IX and X, and innervate the ipsilateral sternocleidomastoid and upper trapezius muscles.

Clinical Aspects   The accessory nerve is tested with a manual muscle test of head rotation (sternocleidomastoid) and shoulder shrug (upper trapezius).

Unilateral lesion of the cranial root (or recurrent laryngeal nerve) produces the following symptoms: The ipsilateral vocal cord becomes fixed and partially adducted, and the voice is hoarse (dysphonia) and reduced to a whisper. Unilateral lesion of the spinal root produces the following symptoms: flaccid paralysis of the sternocleidomastoid with inability to rotate the head to the side opposite the lesion and flaccid paralysis of the upper trapezius with a downward and outward rotation of the scapula.

8 Muscle Physiology

Overview

In spite of its enormous informational processing capacity, the human brain is basically capable of producing only two types of responses: a muscular contraction and a glandular secretion. The contraction of muscle produces the only intrinsic source of force available to stabilize or move body parts in order to produce a desired outcome in the environment. The function of muscle is to transform the stored chemical energy within the body into mechanical work. The motor control system, which is responsible for the controlled application of force, uses muscles as its only effector mechanism. The most distinguishing characteristics of the human motor control system are its versatility and precision.

Three Types of Muscle

Three types of muscles have evolved to perform the different types of work required by the body: smooth, cardiac, and striated. Smooth muscle is found in the walls of the hollow viscera, such as the stomach, circulatory system, and alimentary tract. The contraction time of smooth muscle is slow and well adapted for sustained, rhythmic contractions. When smooth muscle contracts, it produces an emptying of the contents in the visceral organs. For most people, the voluntary control of smooth muscle is restricted to emptying the bowel and bladder. However, rare individuals have demonstrated the ability to voluntarily control some smooth muscle body functions such as blood pressure. Cardiac muscle provides the force behind the central pump of the circulatory system. Smooth muscle and cardiac muscle are controlled by the autonomic nervous system. Striated (skeletal) muscle, the third muscle type, connects bones and produces the force to maintain body posture or cause movement to occur, or both. The body's shape and most of its weight are determined by the bones and the skeletal muscles that move them. Skeletal muscle provides the basis for the voluntary control of human movement.

Structure of Skeletal Muscle

Skeletal muscle consists of bundles (fascicles) of elongated, multinucleated cells called muscle fibers (Fig. 8-1). Each muscle fiber contains bundles of myofibrils that contract in response to neural stimulation. Myofibrils consist of chains of cylindrical units called sarcomeres separated by Z bands. Sarcomeres contain two distinct types of protein: one thick (myosin) and one thin (actin). It is these proteins that give skeletal muscle their striated appearance when viewed under a microscope.

Inside the muscle, individual cells are separated by connective tissue and two distinct systems of tubes are found. Individual muscle fibers are sheathed in connective tissue, endomysium, and collected into bundles by perimysium. Groups of bundles of muscle fibers are joined by epimysium to form skeletal muscles. Within the muscle, capillaries form one system of tubules for delivering blood to the muscle fibers located deep below the surface, and T-tubules form the other system of tubules for delivering the signal and chemicals used in a contraction to the muscle fibers located deep below the surface.

Force and Length Changes Occur Within a Sarcomere

The sarcomere is the contractile unit within the muscle and it is here that force is generated and length change occurs during a muscular contraction. Myosin is located in the center of the sarcomere and actin filaments extend toward the center from either pole, where they are connected to Z bands. Force is generated and movement is produced as myosin heads successively form connections with the actin filament, rotate, break, and re-form connections (sliding filament theory). Length change occurs because the actin filament moves past the myosin, not because either molecule changes its shape. During a concentric contraction actin moves centrally past myosin, during an isometric contraction it is held in place, and during an eccentric contraction actin moves distally. Force and movement are controlled by the hundreds of thousands of connections between actin and myosin (cross bridges) that are formed throughout the muscle.

Three Types of Skeletal Muscle Fibers

Skeletal muscles consist of three types of muscle fiber: slow oxidative (type I), fast oxidative and glycolytic (type IIA), and fast glycolytic (type IIB), which differ in both structural and functional characteristics. Slow oxidative fibers are darker because of high concentrations of myoglobin, sarcoplasm, and mitochondria. Their functional characteristics, including low critical threshold, slow contraction time, low force production, high capacity for oxidative metabolism, and fatigue resistance, make them particularly well suited for the sustained contractions required to maintain posture. Fast glycolytic fibers are the structural and functional antithesis of slow-twitch fibers. Their lighter color comes from low concentrations of myoglobin and granular material. Functional characteristics, such as high critical threshold, fast contraction time, high force production, high capacity for aerobic metabolism, and fast fatigability, make them well suited for

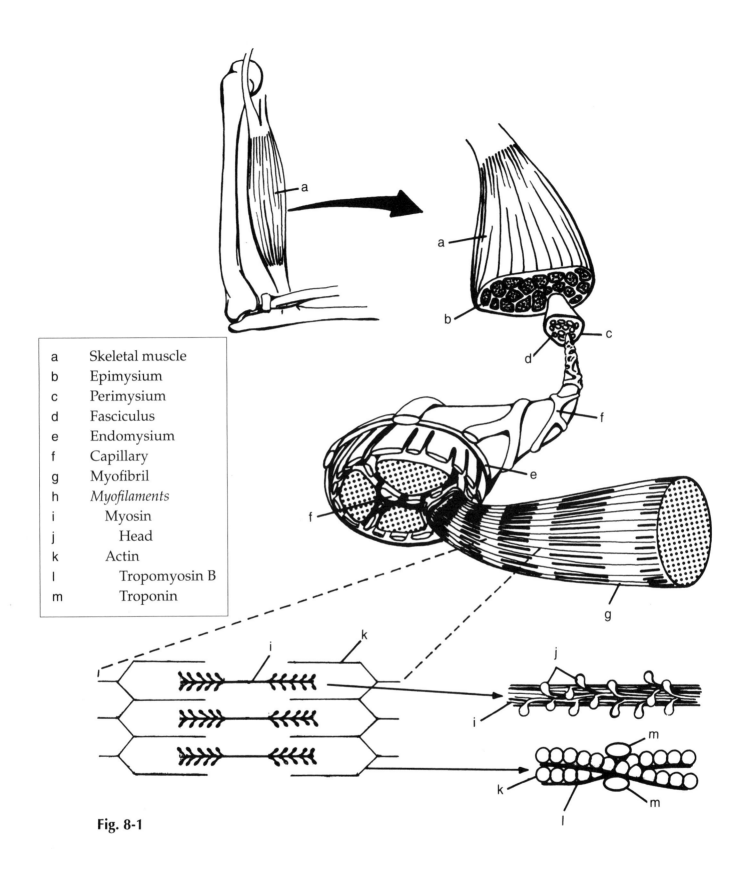

a	Skeletal muscle
b	Epimysium
c	Perimysium
d	Fasciculus
e	Endomysium
f	Capillary
g	Myofibril
h	*Myofilaments*
i	Myosin
j	Head
k	Actin
l	Tropomyosin B
m	Troponin

Fig. 8-1

high force demand, short-duration type tasks. Fast oxidative and glycolytic fibers are intermediate between fast and slow fibers. All skeletal muscles contain all three types of muscle fibers.

Of the two muscles that extend the ankle (soleus and gastrocnemius), the soleus is primarily a postural muscle and the gastrocnemius is mainly a power muscle. Because the line of gravity falls in front of the ankle joint, the maintenance of erect posture requires that an extensor muscle apply continuous force to prevent gravity from pulling the joint into flexion. The soleus muscle with its high percentage of low-threshold, fatigue-resistant, slow-twitch muscle fibers is well adapted to meet these force requirements. To sprint 50 yards or jump from the ground requires a large amount of force to be applied over a short duration. The gastrocnemius muscle with its high percentage of high-force–producing, fast-fatiguing, fast-twitch muscle fibers is well adapted to the high-force, short-duration force requirements of powerful movements.

Muscle fiber type is determined primarily by the frequency of neuronal activity in its axon. Crossed reinnervation of the soleus and gastrocnemius muscles causes marked changes in fiber type profiles and enzymatic activity. Following reinnervation with the soleus nerve, the gastrocnemius muscle develops a much higher percentage of slow-twitch fibers and an increased capacity for aerobic metabolism. Similar reversals in structure and function have been seen in the soleus muscle. In addition to the discharge frequency in the motor neuron, secretion of a "trophic factor" across the myoneural junction may play a role in determining fiber type.

Innervation of Skeletal Muscle

Each skeletal muscle is supplied by one or more nerves. Muscles of the limbs, face, and neck usually receive one nerve and that nerve generally contains fibers from multiple spinal segments. Muscles of the abdominal wall receive innervation from multiple nerves. Nerves usually enter from the deep surface of the muscle along with the blood supply (neurovascular bundle). Muscle nerves contain a wide array of motor and sensory fibers. Motor fibers include large myelinated neurons that innervate skeletal muscle fibers (alpha lower motor neurons), small myelinated neurons that innervate muscle spindles (gamma motor neurons), and nonmyelinated autonomic neurons that innervate vascular smooth muscle (C fibers). Sensory fibers include large-diameter myelinated afferents from muscle spindles and tendon organs (Ia and Ib, respectively) as well as small-diameter, nonmyelinated afferents that supply pain receptors in the connective tissue (C fibers).

Within the muscle, the nerve forms a plexus in the epi- and perimysial septa before entering the endo-mysial spaces around the muscle fibers. Alpha motor neurons branch repeatedly before losing their myelin sheath and terminating on muscle fibers. Each muscle fiber receives a single terminal branch of an alpha motor neuron. The synaptic connection between the neuron and muscle fiber (myoneural or neuromuscular junction) is formed by the motor end plate of the axon and the sole plate on the myofibril. Acetylcholine is the transmitter used at the myoneural junction.

The Functional Unit Within a Skeletal Muscle Is a Motor Unit

Each nerve impulse from a motor neuron produces an obligatory contraction from its muscle fibers (excitation contraction coupling). The individual lower motor neuron and all the muscle fibers that it innervates comprise a motor unit (Fig. 8-2). The motor unit is the smallest functional component with which the motor system controls movement. A muscle's innervation ratio (the number of muscle fibers innervated by a single lower motor neuron) is an indirect index of that muscle's function. Muscles with a high innervation ratio (1:6), such as extraocular muscles and the intrinsic muscles of the tongue, produce little force but have fine control. Muscles with a low innervation ratio (1:2,000), such as the gluteus maximus, produce a great deal of force but lack precise control.

Just as each muscle contains all three types of muscle fibers, each muscle also contains a variety of small, medium, and large motor units. Some muscles, such as extraocular muscles, have more small motor units, whereas others, such as the gluteus maximus, have more large motor units. Small motor units are composed primarily of slow oxidative muscle fibers and are innervated by small-diameter lower motor neurons. Large motor units are composed primarily of fast glycolytic muscle fibers and are innervated by large-diameter lower motor neurons. As force is generated in a muscular contraction, motor units are recruited according to the amount of force they produce. Small motor units (also called fast fatigue resistant) produce the least force, medium motor units (also called slow fatigable) produce intermediate force, and large motor units (also called fast fatigable) produce the most force. The rank order of motor unit recruitment from small to medium to large is called the size principle. The size principle works in reverse for motor unit fatigue, so that large motor units fatigue initially, followed by medium and then small motor units. Thus, small motor units, with their small-diameter lower motor neurons and slow oxidative muscle fibers, are the first to be recruited in a muscular contraction and the last to fatigue. Large motor units are the last to be recruited and provide the greatest force, but their contribution to movement is limited by their fast fatigability.

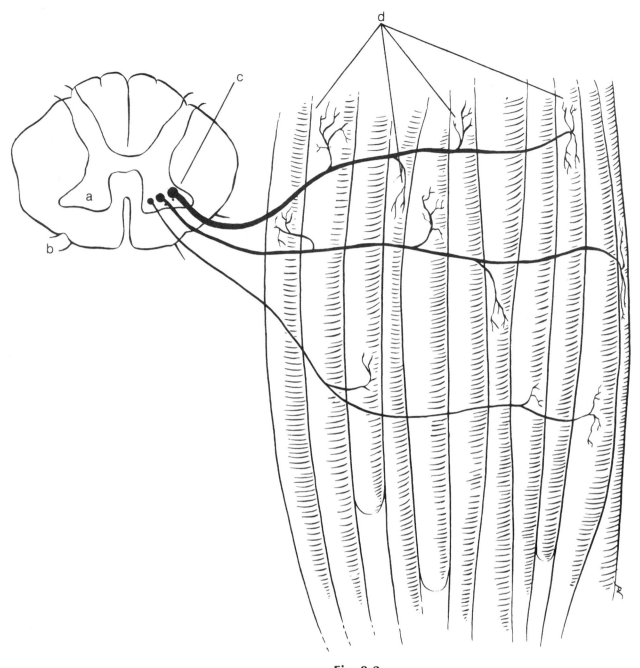

Fig. 8-2

a	Ventral horn
b	Ventral root
c	Lower motor neuron
d	Motor unit

The Force of Muscle Contraction Is Graded in Two Ways

The force of muscle contraction is graded by (1) the orderly recruitment of motor units and (2) modulation of the discharge rate of lower motor neurons. Two physiological principles, the all-or-none principle and the size principle, underlie the orderly recruitment of motor units. According to the all-or-none principle, a motor unit (including all of its muscle fibers) will contract maximally or not at all because once critical threshold is reached at the cell body, a nerve impulse is propagated along the axon and through the telodendria to all muscle fibers of that motor unit. Each muscle fiber responds to the nerve impulse with an obligatory contraction, producing a maximum response from that motor unit. If threshold is not reached, no nerve impulse is generated and no muscular contraction occurs. The second strategy by which the central nervous system can control force production is modulation of the discharge frequency of the alpha motor neuron (rate modulation). Increasing discharge frequency produces increases in contractile force because successive muscular twitches summate.

Recruitment and rate modulation occur together to control the force produced by a muscle contraction. If only a small force is required, only small motor units will be recruited. If a little more force is required, the discharge frequency of lower motor neurons will be increased. If still more force is required, medium and large motor units will be recruited. After all motor units have been recruited and still more force is required, other muscles containing larger motor units can be activated. Such is the case when the gastrocnemius muscle joins the soleus muscle to increase force production in extending the foot at the ankle.

Clinical Aspects

Both the appearance and function of muscle may be affected by disease. Disease may affect the nerve supply to the muscle (neuropathic) or the muscle fibers themselves (myopathic). Examination of the shape, texture, and function of muscle is a normal part of clinical examination. Clinical symptoms of disease of the motor unit include weakness, atrophy, abnormal reflexes, abnormal tone, and involuntary contractions.

Under normal conditions, the strength of a muscle is proportional to its size; for example, an elderly woman has less strength than a young weightlifter, although both have normal muscle function. The loss of muscle bulk (atrophy) occurs for two reasons. Following the loss of innervation, atrophy occurs but weakness is out of proportion to size (neurogenic atrophy). Following lack of use, atrophy occurs but weakness is proportional to the size of the muscle (disuse atrophy). Disuse atrophy is not a sign of disease but neurogenic atrophy is. Atrophy may also occur in myopathic disease and here, too, weakness is usually excessive.

In general, if lower motor neurons are lost, deep tendon reflexes are also lost. Disruption of the reflex arc also results in loss of normal tone or resistance to passive movement. A symptom of upper motor neuron lesion is a rate-dependent increased resistance to passive movement (spasticity). A symptom of lower motor lesion is the absence of resistance to passive movement (flaccid paralysis). Weakness, atrophy, and flaccidity may occur in the trunk or limbs, but it may also occur in the face, tongue, and pharyngeal muscles if the cranial nerves are involved. When this occurs, speech is affected (dysarthria).

Involuntary muscular contractions may or may not indicate disease. Normal muscle shows no electromyographic activity at rest. Denervated muscle exhibits two types of activity at rest. Fibrillations are spontaneous action potentials occurring in single muscle fibers probably due to denervation hypersensitivity at the muscle receptor sites. Fasciculations are thought to represent action potentials involving the entire motor unit and result from diseases of the lower motor neuron such as amyotrophic lateral sclerosis. Poliomyelitis is a disease process that selectively destroys the cell bodies of lower motor neurons, producing weakness (paresis) or paralysis depending on how much of the lower motor neuron pool is involved. Muscle cramps are most often due to a local biochemical imbalance in the muscle after excessive exertion. The "physiological irritability" is usually reversed when biochemical balance is restored. However, prolonged cramping not relieved by rest can indicate an active disease process.

Both the formation and breaking of cross bridges require active energy production (ATP). When ATP is no longer available, the relationship between actin and myosin becomes fixed, which accounts for the rigor mortis seen after death.

9 Control of Voluntary Movement

Overview

Movement is the behavioral result of the organized motor output of the nervous system driving the musculoskeletal system to achieve a particular goal or outcome in the environment. The movement pattern itself can be the goal or it can be a means to achieving some other goal. For example, in gymnastics, dance, and diving, the goal is to produce an ideal movement pattern. In removing your hand from a hot stove, crossing the street, or performing therapeutic exercises, the movement is the means for producing the desired outcome. The only cause of voluntary human movement is the force produced by the contraction of skeletal muscle. While force production forms the biomechanical substrate of movement, it is the careful planning and skillful execution that permit the movement pattern to produce the desired goal. The neurological control of voluntary movement (motor control) is achieved via a functional system that includes components at every level of the nervous system: peripheral, spinal cord, brain stem, and cerebral cortex. Skeletal muscles are innervated by peripheral neurons that originate from motor centers located in the brain stem and spinal cord (lower motor neurons). These centers receive two sources of input, one from sensory neurons originating in the periphery, the other from brain stem and cortical regions that are specialized in the control of movement (upper motor neurons). The spinal cord and brain stem centers control reflexes and simple voluntary movements while the motor areas in the cerebral cortex plan and initiate more complex voluntary movements.

Sensory Information Is Necessary for the Control of Voluntary Movement

Purposeful, goal-directed movement requires a rich, continuous source of sensory feedback. Before initiation of movement, sensory feedback is used to determine the body's position in space and help determine movement parameters. Throughout an ongoing movement, sensory feedback is used to detect and correct movement errors. Thus, sensory information is an integral part of the adaptive, motor control system. The control of ongoing movement requires both internal and external feedback. Internal feedback is provided by proprioceptors in the muscles, joint receptors, and vestibular apparatus, which inform the motor systems about the length and tension of muscles, the angle of joints, and the position of the body in space. External feedback is provided by visual, auditory, and cutaneous receptors on the body surface, which inform the motor systems about the location of objects in space and the body's relation to them.

Skeletal muscle contains two types of proprioceptors, muscle spindles and tendon organs, which keep the central nervous system (CNS) informed about the conditions within the muscle. Muscle spindles are sensitive to changes in muscle length and tendon organs are sensitive to changes in muscle tension. Information about muscle length is critical in allowing the central nervous system to control the position of body parts. Information about muscle tension is essential in controlling the amount of force generated by a muscle.

From outside the muscle, joint receptors provide the remaining type of proprioceptive feedback. Joint receptors consist of specialized nerve endings. which are located in the soft tissue around joints and are sensitive to angular displacement. Joint receptors inform the central nervous system of present joint position, as well as the direction and rate of any change. This information, along with information about muscle length and tension, is critical in guiding the movement if it is to produce the desired outcome.

All three types of proprioceptive information are transmitted into the spinal cord and are ultimately relayed to motor control centers. Information about muscle length and muscle tension is relayed to the cerebellum and then, via the thalamus, to the motor cortex. Information about joint position is relayed first to the thalamus, then to the sensory cortex, and finally to the motor cortex. The motor cortex uses this feedback to plan, initiate, and control the desired movement.

The Trunk and Limbs Are Controlled Independently

In general, the motor control system is designed to provide independent control of the axial and appendicular divisions of the musculoskeletal system. The axial system controls the trunk and proximal limb muscles that provide the postural base for movement. The appendicular system controls the extremities that perform independent manipulation. Independent control of the trunk and extremities is achieved through a series of dual-control systems involving the spinal cord, brain stem, and cortex. The lower motor neurons have their cell bodies located in the ventral horn of the spinal cord. Within the ventral horn the cell bodies of lower motor neurons innervating trunk and proximal limb muscles are located ventromedially while those innervating more distal extremity muscles are located dorsolaterally (Fig. 9-1). Each pool is somatotopically arranged such that the neurons innervating flexor muscles are located dorsally and those innervating extensors are located ventrally. Neurons innervating proximal segments are located medially within the pool while those innervating distal segments are located laterally. Pools of adjacent spinal segments unite to form

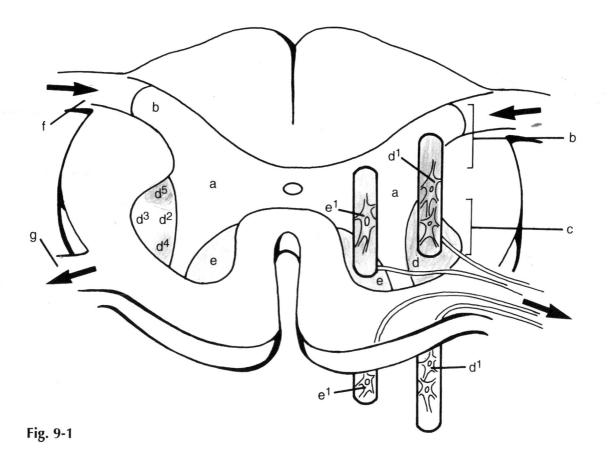

Fig. 9-1

a	Intermediate zone
b	Dorsal horn
c	Ventral horn
d	Dorsolateral cell group
d^1	Motor neurons to limb muscles
d^2–d^5	*Organization of lower motor neuron pool*
d^2	Flexor motor neurons
d^3	Extensor motor neurons
d^4	Proximal limb
d^5	Distal limb
e	Ventromedial cell group
e^1	Motor neurons to axial muscles
f	Dorsal root
g	Ventral root

longitudinal columns of motor neurons that function together to control and coordinate their respective parts. The ventromedial cell group receives supraspinal input from brain stem and cortical motor centers (vestibular nuclei, reticular nuclei, tectum, and motor cortex) via pathways located in the ventromedial portion of the brain stem and spinal cord. The dorsolateral cell group receives supraspinal input from cortical and brain stem motor centers (red nucleus and primary motor cortex) via pathways located in the dorsolateral brain stem and spinal cord.

The Ventromedial System

The ventromedial system (brain stem and cortical motor centers, ventromedial pathways, and ventromedial lower motor neuron pool; Fig. 9-2) controls the posture and balance component of a movement pattern. The medial and lateral vestibulospinal tracts originate from the medial and lateral vestibular nuclei, respectively; descend in the ventral funiculus of the ipsilateral spinal cord; and terminate in the ventromedial cell group. This pathway facilitates the activity of lower motor neurons innervating extensor muscles. The vestibulospinal system uses information from the vestibular receptors (information regarding gravity and acceleration) for the reflex control of the posture and balance components of a movement pattern. The medial and lateral reticulospinal tracts originate from several nuclei in the pontine and medullary portions of the reticular formation, descend in the ventral funiculus of the ipsilateral spinal cord, and terminate in the ventromedial lower motor neuron pool. The reticulospinal system integrates information from the vestibular system and cerebral cortex to help maintain balance. The tectospinal tract originates from the superior colliculus, crosses the midline, and descends in the ventral funiculus only as far as the cervical spinal cord. The tectospinal system integrates input from the cerebral cortex and vestibular system to coordinate movements of the head and eyes. The ventromedial system is phylogenetically older than the dorsolateral system and generally facilitates the activity of lower motor neurons projecting to extensor muscles and inhibits the activity of lower motor neurons projecting to flexors.

The Dorsolateral System

The dorsolateral system (brain stem and cortical motor centers, dorsolateral pathways, and dorsolateral lower motor neuron pool; Fig. 9-3) includes the rubrospinal, corticobulbar, and lateral corticospinal tracts. The dorsolateral system is more than twice as large as the ventromedial system and is responsible for the independent limb, particularly movements involving the hands and feet. The rubrospinal tract (Fig. 9-3) originates from the red nucleus, crosses the midline, descends in the lateral funiculus of the contralateral spinal cord, and terminates in the dorsolateral cell group, where it facilitates the activity of lower motor neurons innervating flexor muscles. Within the limb, the rubrospinal tract has primary responsibility for movements at the more proximal joints.

Descending fibers from the motor cortex have two primary subdivisions, corticobulbar and corticospinal. The corticobulbar tract originates in the motor cortex (areas 8, 4, 6 of Brodmann), descends through the posterior limb of the internal capsule, and terminates on the lower motor neurons of the cranial nerves. Area 8 is the frontal eye field and controls eye movements by way of the oculomotor (III), trochlear (IV), and abducens (VI) cranial nerves. Fibers from areas 4 and 6 control the muscles of the head and face by way of the trigeminal (V), facial (VII), and hypoglossal (IX) cranial nerves. Cortical projections to the trigeminal nucleus are bilateral and approximately equal in strength so that, in most cases, muscles above the eyes cannot be contracted voluntarily on one side only. Cortical projections to the facial and hypoglossal nuclei are also bilateral but contralateral projections are much stronger. Thus, the muscles below the eye can generally be controlled independently, and a lesion of one cerebral hemisphere results in weakness of the contralateral facial and tongue musculature. Fibers from areas 4 and 6 also terminate in the sensory nuclei of the same cranial nerves. These projections help regulate movement-produced sensory feedback.

The corticospinal tract is a massive bundle of fibers, containing approximately one million axons, that originates from the sensorimotor cortex (areas 4, 6, 3, 1, 2; Fig. 9-3). Approximately one third of the fibers originate from the primary motor cortex (area 4), one third from the premotor cortex (area 6), and the remaining third from the somatic sensory cortex (areas 3, 1, and 2). These fibers descend through the posterior limb of the internal capsule, and the vast majority cross the midline in the medulla. Estimates of the portion of the tract that cross the midline vary between 75 and 95 percent. The crossed fibers form the lateral corticospinal tract, descend in the lateral funiculus of the contralateral spinal cord, and terminate in the dorsolateral lower motor neuron pool. The fibers that remain uncrossed form the ventral corticospinal tract.

The ventral corticospinal tract becomes part of the ventromedial projection system because it descends in the ventral funiculus of the ipsilateral spinal cord and terminates in the ventromedial lower motor neuron pools bilaterally (see Fig. 9-2). The bilateral projection occurs at the spinal level of termination. Some fibers terminate in the ipsilateral ventromedial lower motor neuron pool, and some cross the midline to terminate in the contralateral ventromedial lower motor neuron pool. This bilateral projection to motor neurons innervating axial musculature could help provide the trunk stability on which the independent limb manipulation is dependent.

A small percentage of corticospinal tract fibers (estimates range less than 30 percent) terminate on sensory interneurons in the dorsal horn of the spinal cord.

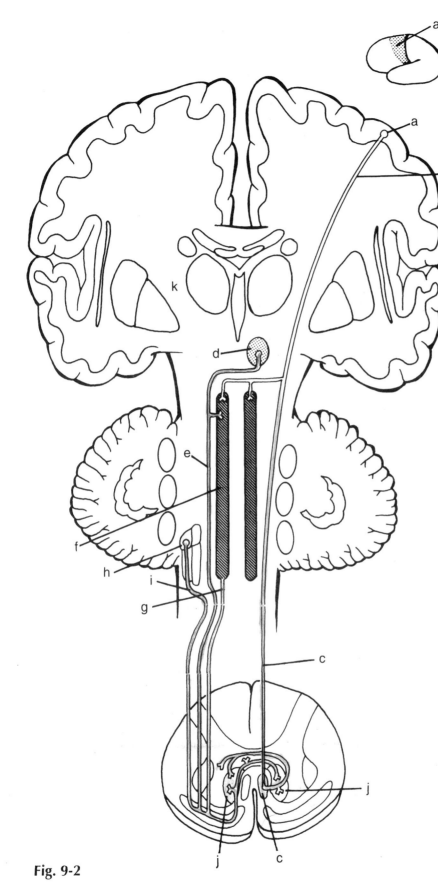

Ventro-medial system

Fig. 9-2

a	Areas 4, 6
b	Upper motor neuron
c	Anterior corticospinal tract
d	Tectum
e	Tectospinal tract
f	Medial reticular formation
g	Reticulospinal tract
h	Lateral vestibular nucleus
i	Vestibulospinal tract
j	Ventromedial lower motor neuron pool
k	Internal capsule

Many of these fibers were the ones that originated from the primary sensory cortex. The synaptic connections formed by these fibers enable the cerebral cortex to influence local reflex activity or modify the sensory input reaching ascending sensory systems. This sensory projection of motor commands could also function in error detection. If sensory neurons were pre-informed of what the movement-produced feedback should look like, any deviation could be identified as a performance error and corrections could begin without further processing delays.

The corticospinal tract was once thought to be responsible for the initiation and control of all "voluntary" movement. It is now known to be concerned primarily with the initiation and control of learned movements of the distal extremities, particularly independent control of the individual digits of the hand, a capacity known as fractionation of movement. This ability is completely and irretrievably lost following lesion of the corticospinal tract.

The corticospinal tract projects to all levels of the spinal cord. The vast majority of fibers form facilitatory polysynaptic connections with lower motor neurons by way of interneurons. A very small percentage of corticospinal tract fibers (estimates range around 3 percent) form monosynaptic connections with lower motor neurons. The discharge rate of corticospinal tract fibers is directly related to the force produced during the movement. Because no other motor system has such a direct association with force production, weakness following neurological insult is a cardinal sign of corticospinal tract involvement.

Table 9-1 is a comparison of ventromedial and dorsolateral systems.

Clinicians often divide the descending pathways into pyramidal and extrapyramidal systems. The pyramidal system consists of the corticospinal fibers that pass through the medullary pyramid and the extrapyramidal system consists of all other descending pathways. This classification system is effective clinically because lesions in the two systems produce distinctively different signs and symptoms.

Serial and Parallel Control Systems

The motor control system, including spinal cord, brain stem, and cortical centers, is organized both in series and in parallel. The serial organization forms a three-level motor control hierarchy; that is, spinal centers are subject to control from the brain stem, which is, in turn, subject to control from the cortex. The loss of hierarchical control is thought to be a mechanism underlying some of the signs and symptoms seen clinically following injury to the CNS (release phenomena). The three motor control centers also function in parallel via the ventromedial and dorsolateral projection systems such that any one center can, to some extent, control movement independent of the other two. The overlapping hierarchical and parallel organization is important in the recovery of function after local lesions.

The lowest level of the motor control hierarchy, the spinal cord, contains neuronal networks (motor centers) that control a variety of reflexes and automatic movements. Spinal motor centers are capable of controlling reflex withdrawal from a noxious stimulus and the alternate activation of flexors and extensors seen in locomotion even after being disconnected from the brain. The middle level of the motor control hierarchy, the brain stem, contains ventromedial and dorsolateral systems that control the motor centers in the spinal cord. The brain stem plays an important part in the regulation of posture and equilibrium by integrating visual and vestibular information with somatosensory input before influencing spinal motor centers. The brain stem is also instrumental in the coordination of head and eye movements. The highest level of the motor control hierarchy consists of three areas of the cerebral cortex: the primary motor cortex, premotor cortex, and supplementary motor cortex. Each area projects directly to spinal motor centers via the corticospinal

Table 9-1   Comparison of Ventromedial and Dorsolateral Systems

Components	Ventromedial System	Dorsolateral System
Tracts	Lateral vestibulospinal Medial vestibulospinal Lateral reticulospinal Medial reticulospinal Tectospinal Ventral corticospinal	Rubrospinal Corticobulbar Lateral corticospinal
Spinal projection	Ventral funiculus	Lateral funiculus
Spinal termination	Ventromedial lower motor neuron pool	Dorsolateral lower motor neuron pool
Body segments	Trunk Proximal limb segments	Distal limb segments
Muscles	+ extensors − flexors	− extensors + flexors
Function	Posture Balance	Skilled (fractionated) movement

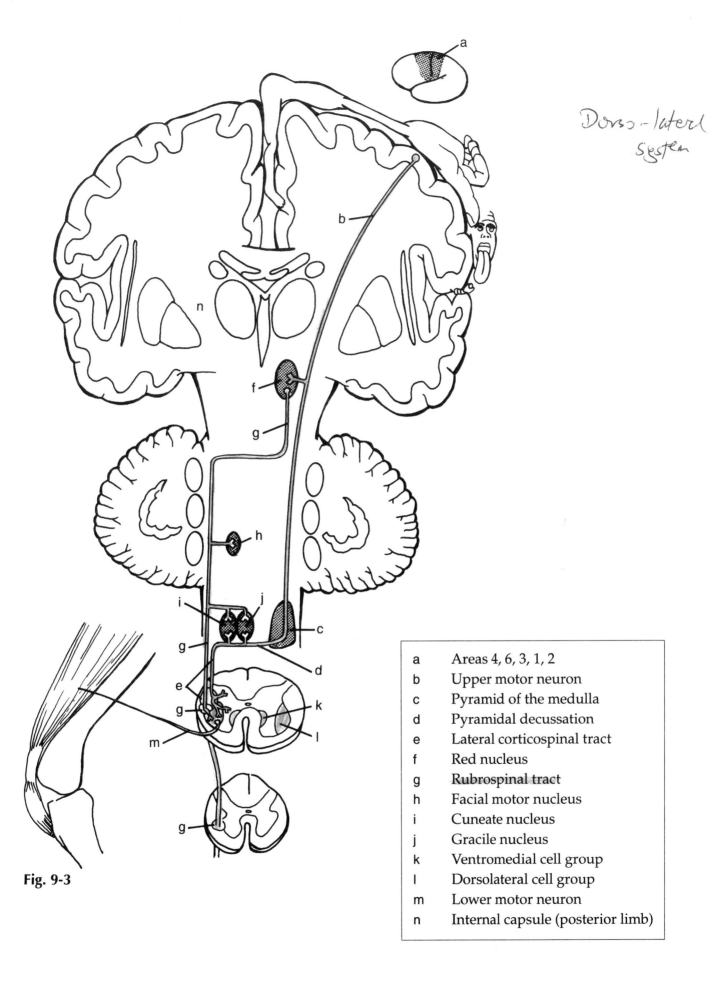

Dorso-lateral
System

a	Areas 4, 6, 3, 1, 2
b	Upper motor neuron
c	Pyramid of the medulla
d	Pyramidal decussation
e	Lateral corticospinal tract
f	Red nucleus
g	Rubrospinal tract
h	Facial motor nucleus
i	Cuneate nucleus
j	Gracile nucleus
k	Ventromedial cell group
l	Dorsolateral cell group
m	Lower motor neuron
n	Internal capsule (posterior limb)

Fig. 9-3

71

tract and indirectly via the brain stem. Premotor and supplementary motor areas receive input from frontal and parietal association areas, project directly to the primary motor cortex, and are involved in the planning and coordination of complex movements.

The structures within each level of the motor control hierarchy are somatotopically arranged; that is, specific areas of that structure are dedicated to the control of particular body parts. This functional organization was discovered when electrical stimulation of a particular site produced a motor response in a specific body part. Somatotopic organization is maintained in all input-output relations (sensory, motor, and interneuronal) such that areas concerned with the control of a particular body part are in communication with one another. Thus, somatotopic organization throughout the system forms a basis for coordinating complex movements among different body parts. The regions that initiate movement of a particular body part are also informed of the sensory consequences of the movement. Each level of the motor control system also receives sensory feedback from the periphery, and by facilitating or inhibiting sensory relay nuclei, higher centers play an active part in determining what information reaches them.

An example of how the system functions to achieve the goal of trunk stabilization is as follows. The supplementary motor and premotor areas concerned with trunk control plan and coordinate co-contractions of the necessary muscles. These areas then inform the trunk region of the primary motor cortex of the necessary actions. The primary motor cortex then activates visual, equilibrium, and righting centers in the brain stem as well as the spinal motor centers controlling the torso. At the spinal level, motor neurons are activated that recruit the motor units which produce the force needed to stabilize the trunk. As the muscles contract, sensory information regarding changes in the visual display or body position with reference to gravity as well as muscle tension, length, and joint position is relayed to the appropriate motor centers. Motor centers then actively choose from the available sensory feedback that which they need to determine if the goal of trunk stability is being achieved or whether some modification of motor commands is necessary.

The Role of the Basal Ganglia and Cerebellum in the Motor Control Hierarchy

The basal ganglia and cerebellum are important subcortical motor centers that function in parallel to help control movement. Because neither structure projects directly onto lower motor neurons, their influence in motor control is indirect. Both structures form subcortical feedback loops by receiving input from the cortex and projecting back to the cortex via the thalamus. However, these feedback loops have important functional differences. First, the basal ganglia project to the supplementary motor and prefrontal areas while the cerebellum projects to the premotor and primary motor areas. Second, the basal ganglia receive input from wider areas of the cerebral cortex than the cerebellum. Third, the basal ganglia receive no direct somatic input from the spinal cord while the cerebellum receives many direct projections from the spinal cord relaying movement-produced changes in sensory feedback. Fourth, the basal ganglia's sole access to lower motor neurons is via the cortex while the cerebellum has other more direct connections via the vestibular nuclei, reticular nuclei, and red nucleus.

As the differences in projections would suggest, the cerebellum seems to be involved in the regulation of specific parameters of movement while the basal ganglia are thought to be involved in more complex aspects of motor planning. The cerebellum acts as a comparator of movement intention (as reflected in cortical output) with movement results (as reflected in the sensory consequences of movement). The cerebellum is responsible for controlling the timing, coordination of synergists, and background tone of a movement. The basal ganglia are responsible for initiating and scaling internally generated movements. Unlike the cerebellum with its primary role in motor control, the basal ganglia also participate in cognitive and limbic-related control systems.

Clinical Aspects

Lesions of the motor control system produce characteristic symptoms that are classified into lower and upper motor neuron syndromes. Lower motor neuron syndrome results from lesions that affect the motor neuron at the level of the cell body (segmental level) or its axon (peripheral level). Lesions to both levels produce the same characteristic symptoms: decreased muscle tone (hypotonia), diminished or absent tendon reflexes (hyporeflexia or areflexia, respectively), muscle weakness (paresis) restricted to a small group of muscles in a segmental or myotomal distribution, fasciculations (involuntary twitching of muscle fascicles), and atrophy (loss of muscle mass). Because of muscle weakness following lower motor neuron lesion, movement patterns tend to include substitution movements, such as the gluteal lurch gait pattern of a patient with polio. Upper motor neuron syndrome is the result of interference with the supraspinal drive (brain stem or cortical levels) of segmental motor centers. Characteristic symptoms include spasticity (velocity-dependent resistance to passive motion), increased tone (hypertonia), and increased deep tendon reflexes (hyperreflexia) in groups of muscles with similar functions. Following upper motor neuron lesion, movement patterns tend to be very stereotypical (pathological synergies), such as the retracted pelvis seen in many individuals following a cerebrovascular accident (CVA). Typically, upper motor neuron syndrome results from a lesion of structures other than the corticospinal tract. The only upper motor neuron lesion that produces weakness is seen in the corticospinal tract.

Motor neuron syndromes may also be produced by lesions of the spinal cord. A hemisection of the spinal cord (Brown-Séquard) has four main clinical consequences. First, lesion of the lateral corticospinal tract produces upper motor neuron symptoms and signs (paralysis, hypertonia, hyperreflexia, positive Babinski, and clonus) on the side of the lesion, generalized below the level of the lesion. Second, lesion of the dorsal and lateral columns produces loss of position sense, vibratory sense, and tactile discrimination on the side of the lesion, generalized below the level of the lesion. Third, lesion of the anterolateral system causes loss of the sensations of pain and temperature on the side opposite the lesion, generalized below the level of the lesion. Fourth, lesion of autonomic fibers produces loss of autonomic functions on the side of the lesion, generalized below the level of the lesion.

The exact symptoms and signs following a lesion will depend on the location of the lesion. The most common cause of lesion in the motor control system is CVA and the most frequently occluded vessels are the middle cerebral artery and the vertebrobasilar system. The abnormal movements that follow a lesion are classified as either negative or positive. Negative signs indicate the loss of particular capacities that were previously controlled by the damaged area, for example, weakness (paresis) or the decreased ability to generate force quickly. Positive signs are stereotypical, involuntary or uncontrolled movements that may occur after lesion. Using a hierarchical model of motor control, positive signs are explained by the withdrawal of the inhibitory influence that the higher center exercised on the lower center that mediates the response. With this reference, positive signs are referred to as release phenomena. Examples of positive signs are hyperactive reflexes or involuntary movements.

As discussed previously, the motor control system is organized both in series and in parallel. This built-in redundancy provides a degree of back-up such that, in the presence of lesion, some degree of the control for a particular movement can be shifted to the remaining systems. However, control is not completely duplicative. In humans, the corticospinal tract provides the only direct descending control over distal limb muscles. These connections endow humans with the unique ability to oppose thumb and index finger tip-to-tip (pincer grip). This ability is completely and irretrievably lost following lesion of the lateral corticospinal tract. Thus, not all results of neurological lesion are reversible.

10 Reflexes

Overview

A reflex response represents the smallest behavioral unit controlled by the nervous system. A reflex is an involuntary and relatively stereotyped response to a specific sensory stimulus. Two features of the sensory stimulus are particularly important in determining a reflex response. First, the location of the stimulus determines where a reflex response will occur. The response is seen in the organ from which the stimulus arose. Second, the strength of the stimulus helps determine the amplitude of the response. A substantial portion of ordinary behavior, including heart rate, respiration, digestion, postural adjustments, and aspects of locomotion, are controlled reflexively. Reflexes are innate and do not require any learning or prior experience to be elicited. The function of a reflex is to produce an automatic response. For example, the withdrawal reflex provides for the automatic removal of a body part that has been injured.

A reflex arc is the neurophysiological unit that controls a reflex response and contains both peripheral and central components. Peripheral components include the effector organ, sensory receptor, and its afferent and efferent neurons. Central components include the synaptic connections between afferent and efferent neurons and any interneurons that may be involved. All somatic reflex connections occur within the central nervous system and all but monosynaptic reflexes (a small percentage of the total) involve interneurons. Polysynaptic reflexes involve one or more interneurons interposed between the afferent and efferent neurons. Reflexes can be classified by the level of the neuraxis where their synapses occur. Those that have their primary synaptic connections contained within a single segmental level of the spinal cord are called segmental reflexes. Those involving more than one segmental level are called intersegmental reflexes and those involving the brain are called supraspinal reflexes. Even a simple reflex response involves many sensory receptors, their afferent neurons, multiple synapses with the interneurons that they recruit, as well as numerous motor units, all of which are integrated into a highly organized and efficient behavioral unit.

Segmental Reflexes

The monosynaptic stretch reflex (myostatic reflex) is the simplest and most commonly cited example of a segmental reflex (Fig. 10-1). Being monosynaptic, it consists of a single sensory neuron, a synapse, and a single motor neuron. One example of a stretch reflex is the patellar (knee-jerk) reflex, which, under testing conditions, begins with a brisk tap on the patellar tendon

that lengthens the quadriceps muscles. The increase in muscle length is sensed by muscle spindles located in the hamstrings, which inform the central nervous system of the rate and extent of the unexpected change in muscle length. The central nervous system then works to correct this perturbation by producing a reflex contraction to return the muscle to its intended length.

The muscle spindle is a proprioceptive receptor that is sensitive to changes in muscle length. It consists of encapsulated fibers (nuclear bag and nuclear chain) located inside skeletal muscle in parallel with the muscle fibers (Fig. 10-1). Information about the rate of change of muscle length is conveyed to the spinal cord by the change in discharge frequency of the muscle spindle primary afferent (Ia). The primary afferent originates from the central (equatorial) region of both nuclear bag and nuclear chain fibers. Information about absolute muscle length is conveyed via secondary afferents (II), which originate predominantly from nuclear chain fibers.

The classic stretch reflex, elicited by a tendon tap, involves the activation of only the muscle spindle primary afferents. Inside the L4 spinal segment, on the same side as the stimulus, the primary afferents establish monosynaptic, facilitatory connection with alpha lower motor neurons, which innervate in the quadriceps muscles. The reflex response is always elicited in the muscle from which the stimulus originated (the homonymous muscle). The tendon tap synchronizes the discharge of all the muscle spindle primary afferents in the quadriceps muscles (approximately 5,000). The synchronized burst of activity across the monosynaptic connections activates several motor units. The reflexively activated motor units produce a concentric contraction intended to return the quadriceps muscles to their previously shorter (resting) length. It is the reflex muscular contraction, attempting to reestablish resting muscle length, that results in the "knee-jerk" response that can be seen after tapping the patellar tendon.

The same reflex control strategy for maintaining a given muscle length underlies the unconscious control of static posture. A given joint position (posture) can be defined by the central nervous system specifying the length in antagonistic pairs of muscles. Maintenance of that position can then be relegated to the stretch reflex mechanisms of antagonistic pairs of muscles, thereby freeing conscious motor control capacity to solve other motor problems.

The simplicity of the reflex mechanism just described is deceiving because the total reflex is much more complex. Not only does the muscle spindle primary afferent establish monosynaptic reflex connections, but it also synapses with ascending fibers, which

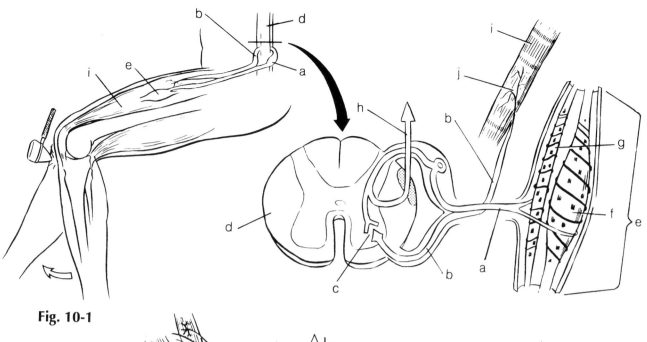

Fig. 10-1

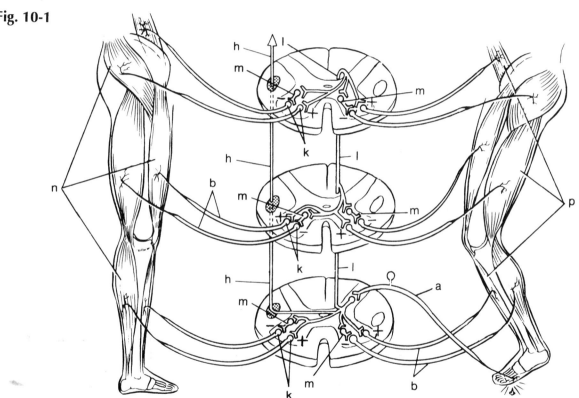

Fig. 10-2

a	Primary sensory afferent	i	Skeletal muscle
b	Alpha lower motor neuron	j	Motor end plate
c	Synapse	k	Reciprocal inhibition
d	Spinal cord	l	Interneuron
e	Muscle spindle	m	Inhibitory interneuron
f	Nuclear bag fiber	n	Extensor muscles
g	Nuclear chain fiber	p	Flexor muscles
h	Ascending neuron		

keep the brain informed about the present condition of the muscles. In addition, the primary afferent synapses with an inhibitory interneuron, which "turns off" the antagonistic muscle group (the hamstrings). The function of the inhibitory connection is to prevent the antagonist from opposing the knee jerk through a reflexive contraction of its own. Inhibition of antagonistic muscle groups is an automatic motor control function that occurs in both voluntary and reflex movements (reciprocal inhibition). Reciprocal inhibition permits coordinated movement between antagonistic pairs of muscles.

Intersegmental Reflexes

The withdrawal reflex is an important self-protection mechanism for removing body parts from harmful situations. Particularly in the case of the lower extremities, where the withdrawal of one leg could jeopardize balance, the withdrawal reflex is coupled with a crossed extensor reflex (Fig. 10-2). When the flexor muscles of one leg are activated and the leg is withdrawn, there is a simultaneous reflex activation of the extensors of the opposite leg. This reflex coupling or coactivation prevents an individual from falling when the injured leg is withdrawn. The pain-sensing fibers in the withdrawn leg activate propriospinal neurons (interneurons that remain within the spinal cord) that in turn activate flexor muscles for all three joints of the lower extremity. Because the hip receives innervation from segmental levels as high as L1 and the ankle as low as S2, the propriospinal neurons must transmit the reflex signal across many levels of the spinal cord. In addition to activating the flexor muscles of one entire extremity, propriospinal neurons also activate the extensor muscles of the opposite extremity. By crossing to the opposite side of the spinal cord and activating the appropriate extensor muscles (which also receive innervation from several segmental levels), the propriospinal neurons enable body weight to be transferred from the leg being withdrawn to the leg being extended. Further, appropriate reciprocal inhibition is an integral part of this reflex-coupling matrix and ensures that both flexion and extension movements will be unopposed by antagonistic muscles.

Neural networks within the spinal cord including interneurons and propriospinal neurons are capable of generating meaningful motor output. These neural networks or central pattern generators play an important part in the control of locomotion. The reciprocal pattern of muscular contractions that produce the stance and swing phases of the gait cycle is controlled by spinal pattern generators. The activity of spinal pattern is modulated by peripheral afferent neurons from muscle, joints and cutaneous receptors, local spinal circuits, and descending pathways. Under predictable, undisturbed conditions, spinal pattern generators permit the reflex control of locomotion in the absence of constant supraspinal vigilance.

Supraspinal Reflexes

The class of reflexes known as righting reactions has a long central loop that passes through the midbrain. Their peripheral mechanisms, both sensory and motor, are the same as spinal reflexes; however, in this case, interneurons ascend to the level of the midbrain (Fig. 10-3). The purpose of righting reactions is to keep the body oriented in space. As the body is tilted, the head is adjusted so as to remain vertically aligned with the pull of gravity and to keep the eyes horizontal. Head-body alignment is critical in maintaining spatial orientation. The vestibular receptors located in the inner ear sense the change in body position and relay this information to the vestibular nuclei in the medulla. From the brain stem, the information is sent to the midbrain, where it is integrated with other sensory information (visual, tactile, and proprioceptive) regarding the change in body position. An appropriate reflex response that will maintain the vertical alignment of the head is achieved by activating the motor units that produce the necessary muscular contractions.

The description given here of the classes of reflexes has been simplified, for even the simplest reflexes involve hundreds of thousands of sensory neurons, interneurons, and motor units. Since reflexes always occur against a background of ongoing activity in the nervous system, they have a dynamic quality and are not completely predictable on the basis of stimulus input alone. The condition or state of the central nervous system, within which the synaptic events occur, will have an effect on the behavioral response that is produced.

Central Control of the Reflex Arc

Supraspinal influence on segmental levels of the spinal cord is transmitted via descending tracts and manifested in one of two ways. If supraspinal influences are strong enough to reach threshold, motor neurons will discharge and the effector apparatus will respond. However, if supraspinal influence does not reach threshold, the ongoing level of background activity will fluctuate momentarily and then return to a resting level. Clear understanding of the ongoing fluctuation of neuronal activity requires that the oversimplified cell-to-cell concept of the organization of the nervous system be replaced by the more realistic concept of populations of cells.

The discharge zone consists of those postsynaptic cells (in the population) that reach threshold and discharge. The subliminal fringe includes those postsynaptic cells surrounding the discharge zone that are partially depolarized but do not reach threshold. The size of both the discharge zone and subliminal fringe is proportional to the afferent input. Thus, if either the number of afferent fibers or the frequency of impulses increases, more cells from the subliminal fringe may be recruited into the discharge zone. As additional recruitment occurs, a new and larger subliminal fringe is

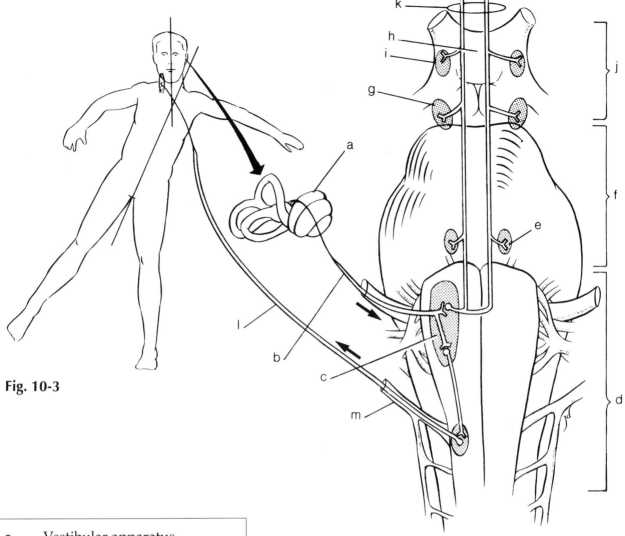

Fig. 10-3

a	Vestibular apparatus
b	Eighth cranial nerve
c	Vestibular nuclei
d	*Medulla*
e	Sixth cranial nerve nuclei
f	*Pons*
g	Fourth cranial nerve nuclei
h	Optic chiasm
i	Third cranial nerve nuclei
j	*Midbrain*
k	Medial longitudinal fasciculus
l	Alpha lower motor neuron
m	Spinal accessory nerve
n	Sensory neuron
p	Interneuron
q	Discharge zone
r	Subliminal fringe
s	Overlapping fringe

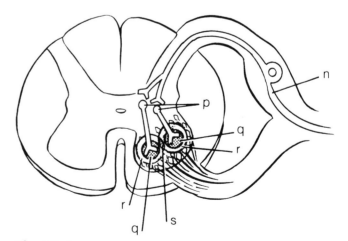

Fig. 10-4

created. Also, the subliminal fringes from adjacent discharge zones may overlap, causing additional cells to reach threshold and become incorporated into the discharge zone (spatial summation).

The gray matter of the spinal cord consists of the cell bodies of neurons that are packed as tightly as possible (thousands per square centimeter). The ventral horn contains one example of a population (pool) of cells: the cell bodies of lower motor neurons. For a single lower motor neuron to reach threshold, it requires almost synchronous discharge of 50 to 100 facilitatory synapses (convergence). Before this can occur, the incoming sensory afferents must divide and subdivide, recruiting the necessary interneurons (divergence). Each volley of afferent impulses fractionates the population of postsynaptic cells into a discharge zone and a subliminal fringe (Fig. 10-4).

Clinical Aspects

Evaluation of reflex responses is a normal part of clinical examination. Both superficial and deep reflexes are included in the neurological portion of a clinical examination. Superficial reflexes (abdominal and cremasteric) provide a means of indirect evaluation of sensory receptors located in the skin, their afferent and efferent neurons, and the level of the neuraxis where synaptic connections occur. Deep tendon reflexes provide a means of indirect evaluation of muscle spindles, their afferent neurons, the segmental level of the neuraxis within which the synapses are located, and motor units from the muscle where the reflex response occurs.

In general, both upper and lower motor neuron syndromes include reflex abnormalities. In upper motor neuron syndrome, superficial (cutaneous) reflexes are reduced (hyporeflexia) while deep tendon reflexes are exaggerated (hyperreflexia). Specifically, abdominal and cremasteric reflexes (superficial reflexes) are diminished or absent on the side of the lesion while deep tendon reflexes are hyperactive. Babinski's sign (dorsiflexion of the great toe and fanning of the other toes in response to an uncomfortable stimulation of the sole of the foot) and clonus (repetitive stretch reflex–induced jerking of a muscle) are both positive in the presence of upper motor neuron lesion. In lower motor neuron syndrome, both superficial and deep tendon reflexes are absent (areflexia). Significant variations occur in reflex responsiveness between individuals and within the same individual on repeated testing. The primary focus for the clinical interpretation of reflex responsiveness is bilateral asymmetry within a given individual, not comparison between individuals.

The primary function of the visceral nervous system is to maintain the environment inside the body within physiological limits (homeostasis). Homeostasis is maintained through the unconscious reflex regulation of smooth muscle, cardiac muscle, and glands by the autonomic nervous system. In the presence of a cervical spinal cord lesion, the ability to reflexively regulate arterial blood pressure when tilted and to maintain a stable body temperature is lost. Also, bladder distention or innocuous skin stimulation in these individuals may trigger a potentially life-threatening reflex response that includes massive sympathetic excitation that produces intense sweating, muscle and skin vasoconstriction, tachycardia, and hypertension (automatic dysreflexia).

11 *Sensory Systems*

Overview

The function of the sensory system is to provide the central nervous system with the information necessary to regulate behavior. This information comes from three broad categories: the external world, the internal environment, and the position of the body in space. Sensory input is also essential in maintaining arousal within the nervous system. Information in the form of energy changes (mechanical, thermal, or photic) is detected by specialized sensory receptors and transmitted to the central nervous system for interpretation. Some sensory information reaches consciousness and is used in the decision-making process while much more is processed subconsciously.

The sensory system can be subdivided into four functional categories: general somatic afferent (GSA), which consists of sensory information from skin, skeletal muscle, and joints; general visceral afferent (GVA), which consists of sensory information from viscera and smooth muscle that rarely reaches consciousness; special somatic afferent (SSA), which consists of sensory information regarding vision, audition, and equilibrium; and special visceral afferent (SVA), which consists of sensory information regarding taste and smell. The following discussion focuses primarily on general somatic sensory information.

General Organization of Somatic Sensory Systems

The somatic sensory system contains three primary components: receptor organs, sensory pathways, and brain centers. All three components are specialized for the individual modalities of the somatic sensory system (touch-pressure, position, thermal, and pain). Receptor organs (sensory receptors) are specialized components of the peripheral nervous system that detect and convert changes in various energy forms (mechanical, thermal, chemical, and photic) into electrical potentials and report that information to the central nervous system. Individual modalities utilize specialized sensory pathways along which their specific type of information is transmitted to centers within the central nervous system where that form of information is interpreted (perceived). At the level of the cerebral cortex, information from individual modalities is integrated to construct an image of what is occurring in the "outside world."

Specialized receptors, central pathways, and brain centers are organized into functional sensory systems. Sensory systems have both a hierarchical and parallel organization. Hierarchical organization means that sensory information is transmitted sequentially via several orders of neurons located in relay nuclei and is processed at each relay station under the control of higher stations in the system. Parallel organization means that individual modalities are served by separate, parallel systems and that a given sensory modality, like touch, can be transmitted by more than one system at the same time. Parallel organization of sensory systems accounts for why some functional ability may remain after a primary sensory system has been destroyed.

In general, somatic sensory systems consist of a three-neuron projection system (Fig. 11-1). First-order neurons extend from the sensory receptor into the central nervous system. The cell bodies of first-order neurons are located in dorsal root ganglia if they innervate receptors located in the body or in cranial nerve nuclei if they innervate receptors located in the head. The axons of first-order neurons bifurcate into peripheral and central branches. The peripheral branch innervates receptor organs and constitutes the sensory component of peripheral nerves. The central branch enters the central nervous system via the dorsal roots of spinal nerves or the sensory component of cranial nerves. Second-order neurons transport the information from first-order neurons to the thalamus on the opposite side (contralateral). The cell bodies of second-order neurons are located in the dorsal horn of the spinal cord or in relay nuclei in the medulla. The axons of second-order neurons cross the midline (decussate) and are grouped into tracts (fasciculi) located in the white matter of the spinal cord (funiculi). In the brain stem, the axons of second-order neurons continue to ascend in tracts (referred to as lemnisci) and terminate by synapsing with third-order neurons located in specific sensory nuclei in the thalamus. The axons of third-order neurons project to the primary somatosensory cortex located in the postcentral gyrus (areas 3, 1, and 2 of Brodmann) of the parietal lobe. Throughout the entire three-neuron projection system, somatic sensory systems maintain a somatotopic organization such that the surface of the body is represented in a topographic fashion in the pathways, relay nuclei, and the primary sensory cortex.

Part of the general organization of sensory systems includes the establishment and organization of a zone through which dorsal root fibers enter the spinal cord. Before entry, large-diameter, myelinated axons, such as those from proprioceptors, are grouped so that they enter the spinal cord medially (Fig. 11-2). Medium-diameter myelinated axons, such as those mediating tactile sense, enter the spinal cord as the middle group. Small-diameter, unmyelinated axons, such as those mediating pain and temperature, enter the spinal cord as the lateral group.

a	Sensory receptor
b	*First-order neuron*
b¹	Distal axon
b²	Cell body
b³	Proximal axon
c	*Second-order neuron*
c¹	Cell body
c²	Axon
d	*Third-order neuron*
d¹	Cell body
d²	Axon
e	Thalamus
f	Primary sensory cortex
g	Sensory homunculus
h	Dorsal root entry zone
h¹	Large-diameter fibers
h²	Medium-diameter fibers
h³	Small-diameter fibers
i–j	*Dorsal columns*
i	Fasciculus gracilis
i¹	Sacral
i²	Lumbar
j	Fasciculus cuneatus
j¹	Thoracic
j²	Cervical
k	Dorsal spinocerebellar tract
l	Ventral spinocerebellar tract
m	Anterolateral system
m¹	Sacral
m²	Lumbar
m³	Thoracic
m⁴	Cervical
n	Ventral spinothalamic tract

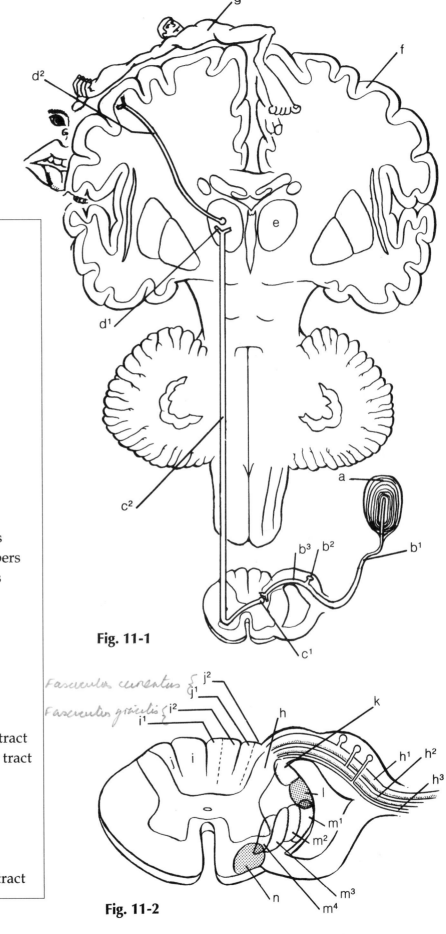

Fig. 11-1

Fig. 11-2

Receptors: General Organization and Mechanisms

Receptor mechanisms of the sensory system consist of nonneural and neural tissue. In many cases (such as the eye, ear, muscle spindle, and hair cells) the nonneural support structure forms the bulk of the receptor organ. The nonneural tissue provides support, focuses, and amplifies energy changes onto the neural tissue. For example, in the case of the hair cell, which functions as a lever arm, mechanical deformations are sensed, amplified, and focused on the nerve ending that is wrapped around the base of the hair follicle.

The neural portion of the receptor organ is formed by the distal segment of a first-order neuron. A single primary sensory afferent and all the sensory receptors it innervates constitute a sensory unit. The number of sensory receptors within a given area of body surface is the receptor density. The peripheral region from which a stimulus activates a central neuron is the sensory field of that neuron. The sensory field for most central sensory neurons has a center-surround organization such that an adequate stimulus applied in the center of the receptive field causes the neuron to increase discharge frequency while a corresponding stimulus applied in the surround area causes a reduction in discharge frequency. The size of sensory fields varies in different parts of the body. The areas with the greatest sensory discrimination, such as the finger tips and mouth, have high receptor density and the receptors have small receptive fields. Somatotopic representation within sensory systems is proportional to sensitivity. Thus, somatotopic representations are distorted such that the areas with the greatest sensitivity have the greatest representation. One example of this organization is the homunculus of the primary somatosensory cortex, with its large representation of face, hands, and feet, and proportionately smaller representation of extremities and trunk (see Fig. 11-1).

Under the right circumstances, nerve impulses can be generated by the nerve tissue within the receptor organ. Although the mechanism by which receptor potentials are produced varies with the type of receptor organ, certain general principles of receptor physiology are common to all. Presentation of an adequate stimulus (specialized energy source of sufficient intensity) produces a local change in nerve membrane permeability (generator potential). The magnitude of the generator potential is graded in response to stimulus intensity, and if the generator potential reaches threshold, an action potential is initiated. The magnitude of the generator potential and therefore the magnitude of the stimulus are encoded in the frequency of action potentials (discharge frequency). Because receptors have thresholds, they act as the first level of analysis for sensory information. If stimulus intensity is subthreshold, no nerve impulse is generated. Receptor sensitivity is controlled by feedforward mechanisms from the central nervous system. This ensures that neither the central nervous system nor the organism is the passive recipient of sensory information from the environment.

Specialized receptor types have evolved such that a given receptor is more sensitive (has a lower threshold) to one particular type of energy change. Anatomical structure is the primary factor accounting for receptor specialization. Based on adequate stimulus, sensory receptors can be classified into chemoreceptors (olfaction, taste), mechanoreceptors (touch and pressure receptors, muscle spindles, tendon organs, labyrinthine hair receptors), thermal receptors, and photoreceptors (vision; Fig. 11-3).

Receptor Adaptation

Regardless of receptor type, the frequency with which it discharges is a function of stimulus intensity and duration. However, if a stimulus of constant intensity is applied over a long time period, discharge frequency does not remain constant. Discharge frequency is highest at initial stimulus presentation and decreases gradually over time (receptor adaptation). The nervous system is concerned primarily with changes in energy form. When stimulus intensity remains constant, the discharge frequency from the sensory receptor reflects the diminishing informational content of the stimulus. Different receptor types are better adapted to transmit unique types of information because some receptors adapt quickly whereas others adapt more slowly. For example, fast-adapting receptors (pacinian and Meissner's corpuscles) respond primarily to stimulus intensity, and, therefore, they react maximally while the stimulus change is actually occurring. The bursts of response frequency relate to the rate and magnitude of stimulus change. This type of receptor acts as a graded, on/off switch informing the central nervous system about onset, offset, and rate of energy changes. Slowly adapting receptors (Merkel's receptors and Ruffini's corpuscles) respond primarily to continued stimulus application. They keep the central nervous system constantly apprised of the status of the body and its relationship with its surroundings.

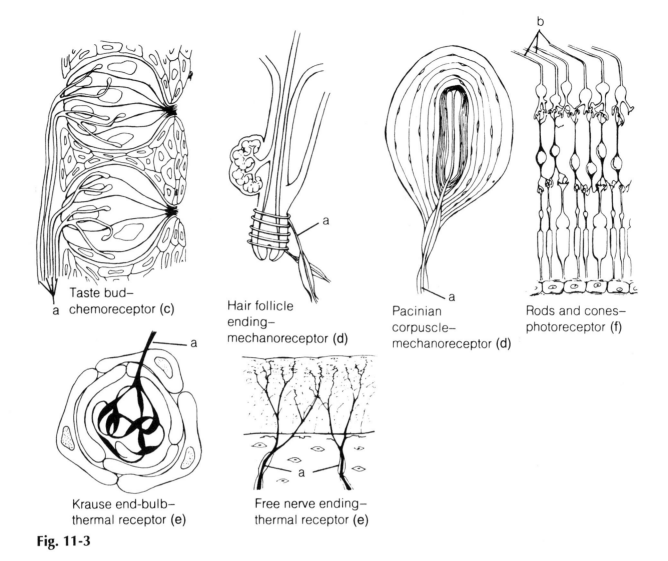

Taste bud–
a chemoreceptor (c)

Hair follicle
ending–
mechanoreceptor (d)

Pacinian
corpuscle–
mechanoreceptor (d)

Rods and cones–
photoreceptor (f)

Krause end-bulb–
thermal receptor (e)

Free nerve ending–
thermal receptor (e)

Fig. 11-3

a	First-order sensory neuron
b	Second-order neuron
c	Chemoreceptor
d	Mechanoreceptor
e	Thermal receptor
f	Photoreceptor

Major Sensory Pathways

Somatic sensory information is conveyed along two major ascending systems in the spinal cord: dorsal column–medial lemniscal system and anterolateral system. The spinocerebellar tracts convey proprioceptive information from the body to the cerebellum but cannot be tested clinically and so are not discussed here.

Pathway for Tactile Discrimination and Arm Proprioception (Dorsal Column–Medial Lemniscal Pathway)

Tactile discrimination (touch and vibration sense) is subserved by low threshold mechanoreceptors located in the skin (hair cells; Merkel's receptors; Meissner's, Ruffini's, and pacinian corpuscles), and limb proprioception is subserved by low threshold mechanoreceptors located in joints, tendons, and muscles (joint receptors, tendon organs, and muscle spindles).

The cell bodies of first-order neurons are located in the dorsal root ganglia, with distal axons projecting from mechanoreceptors and proximal axons projecting into the spinal cord via the medial division of the dorsal root entry zone (Fig. 11-4). After entry, the first-order neurons ascend uninterrupted in the ipsilateral dorsal columns to the brain stem. The dorsal columns also contain a smaller percentage of axons from second-order neurons that originated in laminae III and IV of the dorsal horn. The dorsal columns are located in the posterior funiculus and consist of the fasciculus gracilis and fasciculus cuneatus (see Fig. 11-2). The fasciculus gracilis lies adjacent to the posterior medial septum and contains fibers from the ipsilateral sacral, lumbar, and lower thoracic segments. The fasciculus cuneatus includes fibers from the upper thoracic and cervical segments. It exists only from T6 and above, where it is located lateral to the fasciculus gracilis in the posterior funiculus. Therefore, the dorsal columns are organized somatotopically. First-order neurons contained in the dorsal columns terminate in the dorsal column nuclei (nucleus gracilis and nucleus cuneatus) located at the base of the medulla. The cell bodies of second-order neurons are located in these nuclei and the axons cross the midline and project to the ventral posterolateral nucleus (VPL) of the contralateral thalamus via the medial lemniscus. Third-order neurons project from the thalamus to the primary sensory cortex via the posterior limb of the internal capsule.

Proprioceptive information traveling in this system originates primarily from the upper extremities and face, but the lower extremities are also represented. From the upper extremity, proprioceptive information travels in the same pathway as tactile information: Axons in the fasciculus cuneatus synapse with neurons in a specialized portion of the nucleus cuneatus, whose axons project in the contralateral medial lemniscus.

From the nucleus cuneatus, proprioceptive information from the upper extremity also projects to the cerebellum via the cuneocerebellar tract. From the lower extremity, most proprioceptive information is projected to the cerebellum via Clarke's nucleus and the dorsal spinocerebellar tract. In the caudal medulla second-order neurons synapse with neurons that join the contralateral medial lemniscus. From the face, first-order proprioceptive neurons, traveling in the trigeminal nerve, synapse in the pons with second-order neurons that join the contralateral medial lemniscus. Within the ventral posterior nucleus of the thalamus, proprioceptive input from the trunk and limbs terminates on cells in the lateral division (VPL) while input from the face terminates on cells in the medial division (VPM).

The dorsal column–medial lemniscal pathway is necessary for tactile discrimination (stereognosis) and the ability to distinguish two separate points applied to the skin simultaneously (two-point discrimination), and to distinguish an object's size, weight, and texture in the hand, as well as to recognize numbers and letters drawn on the skin (stereognosis). Other behaviors supported by this pathway include the ability to determine and replicate body position and the ability to perceive vibration. An essential anatomical feature that helps to support the discriminative and localization functions of the dorsal column–medial lemniscal system is the somatotopic organization found at each level of the system.

Clinical Aspects Symptoms produced by lesions of the dorsal column–medial lemniscal pathway are manifest primarily as defects in joint position sense and stereognosis. Diffuse involvement of large-diameter neurons causes loss of tactile discrimination and inability to detect joint position and vibration, which produces extreme difficulty in manipulating objects without visual guidance. These lesions also cause loss of muscle coordination and severe disturbances of locomotion because of loss of proprioception (sensory ataxia). The dorsal column system provides fast, accurate feedback about movement, and coordinated motor output suffers from lesions at any level of this system.

Because of redundancy and parallel pathways for transmission of tactile and proprioceptive information, central lesions of the dorsal column system produce less severe or partial abnormalities. Because the system is uncrossed until the medulla, lesions in the peripheral or spinal levels, up to and including the nuclei, produce symptoms on the side of the lesion. Lesions of the medial lemniscus, thalamus, or sensory cortex will produce similar symptoms but on the side opposite the lesion.

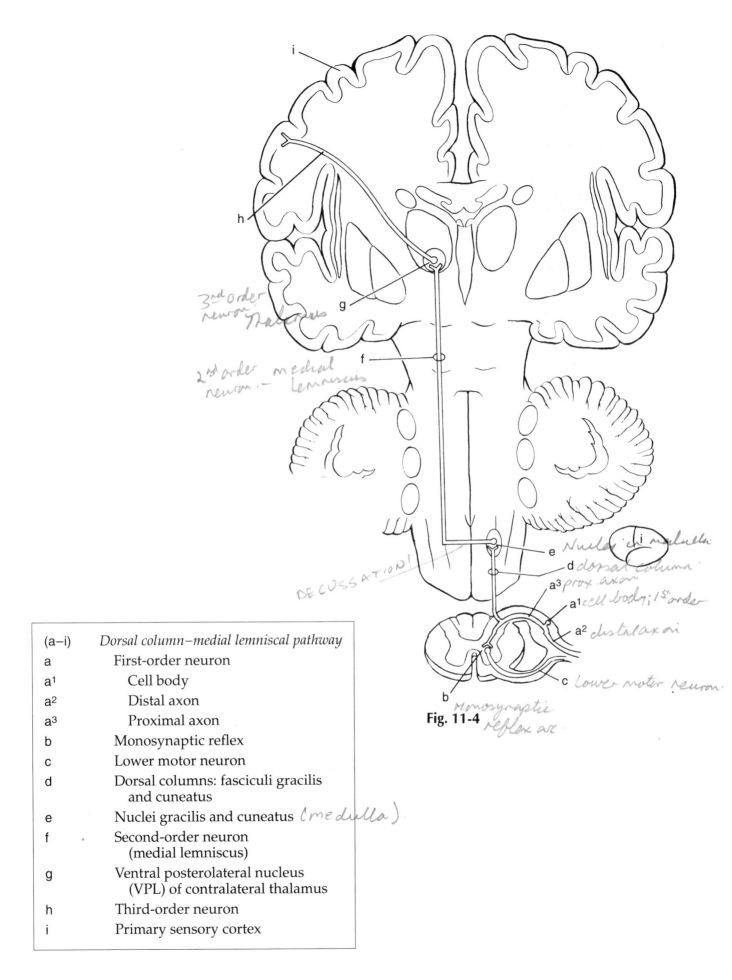

Handwritten annotations on figure:
- 3rd order neuron, Thalamus
- 2nd order neuron — medial lemniscus
- DECUSSATION!
- e Nuclei in medulla
- d dorsal column
- a³ prox. axon
- a¹ cell body; 1st order
- a² distal axon
- c Lower motor neuron
- b monosynaptic reflex arc

Fig. 11-4

(a–i)	*Dorsal column–medial lemniscal pathway*
a	First-order neuron
a¹	Cell body
a²	Distal axon
a³	Proximal axon
b	Monosynaptic reflex
c	Lower motor neuron
d	Dorsal columns: fasciculi gracilis and cuneatus
e	Nuclei gracilis and cuneatus (medulla)
f	Second-order neuron (medial lemniscus)
g	Ventral posterolateral nucleus (VPL) of contralateral thalamus
h	Third-order neuron
i	Primary sensory cortex

Pathway for Pain and Temperature (Lateral Spinothalamic Tract)

Information about pain and temperature from the opposite side of the body is transmitted in the anterolateral system (neospinothalamic and paleospinothalamic tracts). The anterolateral system also carries tactile and proprioceptive information. Because of this functional overlap, individuals with a lesion in the dorsal columns retain some crude tactile and proprioceptive sensibility.

The complex phenomenon referred to as pain can be subdivided into fast or direct pathway and slow or indirect pathway. The two types of pain have different receptors, central pathways, and cortical projection regions. Fast or direct pain is conveyed by the neospinothalamic system and slow or indirect pain is conveyed by the paleospinothalamic system.

Fast or direct pain is sharp, well localized, and short-lived, and usually does not require a clinic visit for pain relief. This type of pain is sensed by high threshold mechanoreceptors innervated by small myelinated axons (A delta fibers; Fig. 11-5). The proximal axon of first-order neurons enters the spinal cord in the intermediate division of the dorsal root entry zone and joins with the tract of Lissauer. Fibers from the tract of Lissauer divide into short ascending and descending branches (one or two levels from the level of entry) and synapse with second-order neurons located in the ipsilateral dorsal horn (laminae I and V). Axons of second-order neurons cross the midline in the anterior gray and white commissures and ascend as the neospinothalamic tract, which synapses on third-order neurons located in the VPL of the thalamus. Axons of third-order neurons project to the primary sensory cortex. This system is somatotopically organized throughout (fibers that convey thermal information are located anterior to those that convey information about noxious stimuli), and well adapted for localizing the source of the noxious stimulus.

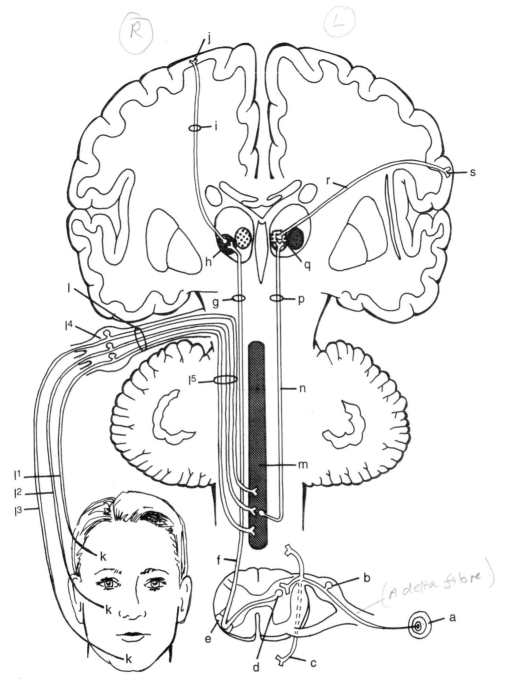

Fig. 11-5

	FAST/DIRECT. PAIN	l	Trigeminal nerve (V)
a	Pain receptor (mechanoreceptor)	l¹	Ophthalmic division
b	First-order neuron *D.R.G.*	l²	Maxillary division
c	Dorsolateral tract of Lissauer	l³	Mandibular division
d	Substantia gelatinosa	l⁴	Gasserian ganglion
e	Spinothalamic tract	l⁵	Descending spinal tract of V
f	Second-order neuron	m	Spinal nucleus of V
g	Lateral lemniscus	n	Second-order neuron
h	VPL of contralateral thalamus	p	Medial lemniscus
i	Third-order neuron	q	VPM of contralateral thalamus
j	Primary sensory cortex (body region)	r	Third-order neuron
k–s	*Pain and temperature from face*	s	Primary sensory cortex (face region)
k	Pain receptor (mechanoreceptor)		

Slow or indirect pain is a diffuse, dull aching or burning sensation that outlasts the stimulus and drives people to the clinic seeking pain relief (analgesia). This type of pain is sensed by polymodal nociceptive receptors innervated by small-diameter, unmyelinated neurons (C fibers; Fig. 11-6). The proximal axon of first-order neurons enters the spinal cord in the medial division of the dorsal root entry zone, joins with the tract of Lissauer, and synapses with second-order neurons located in the ipsilateral dorsal horn (lamina V). Axons of second-order neurons cross the midline in the anterior gray and white commissures and ascend as the paleospinothalamic tract. In the brain stem, second-order neurons synapse in the reticular formation of the medulla and pons, the midbrain, and two thalamic nuclei. Neurons in the reticular formation relay information to the thalamus and other diencephalic structures. Midbrain projections (spinomesencephalic tract) terminate primarily in the superior colliculus and periaqueductal gray (the area surrounding the cerebral aqueduct). This area contains neurons that are part of a descending pathway that regulates pain transmission by releasing analgesic transmitter substances into the dorsal horn. Thalamic projections include the intralaminar and posterior nuclei. Neurons from the intralaminar nuclei project to the basal ganglia and cortical areas associated with the limbic system. The limbic system is concerned with the control of drive, motivation, and affect. The posterior nuclei project to regions of the parietal lobe outside the primary sensory cortex. The reticular projections are what allow the paleospinothalamic system to increase arousal levels. The limbic projections are what give the noxious stimulus or the response to it an affective component (making a face, cursing, crying, or even vomiting). The paleospinothalamic system is not somatotopically organized, which explains why patients have difficulty localizing the source of pain.

The pain and thermal pathway from the head has first-order neurons with cell bodies located in the gasserian (semilunar) ganglion of the trigeminal nerve (V). The cell bodies of second-order neurons are located in the spinal nucleus of the trigeminal nerve and project to the VPM nucleus of the contralateral thalamus. Third-order neurons project from the thalamus to the primary sensory cortex in the posterior limb of the internal capsule (see Fig. 11-5).

Clinical Aspects Symptoms produced by lesions of the anterolateral system vary according to the level of the neuraxis involved. Lesions outside the nervous system frequently stimulate adjacent free nerve endings, thereby producing the subjective sensation of pain. This symptom is most important in calling attention to pathological processes occurring in internal organs, most of which contain no pain receptors of their own. Lesions that involve the peripheral level may cause either the sensation of pain when involving nonneural tissue or the loss of pain and temperature sensibility in the area subserved by the affected nerves. Lesions of the central nervous system that involve the anterolateral system result in an inability to perceive pain or discriminate hot from cold on the contralateral side of the body below the level of the lesion. At the level of the brain stem, lesions produce loss of pain and temperature sensibility in the contralateral body and ipsilateral face. A lesion that affects the ventral posterior thalamic nucleus causes a complete loss of all general somatic sensory information from the contralateral face, trunk, and limbs. Thalamic lesions sometimes produce a severe burning pain in the area of sensory loss.

The differences in the functional organization of the dorsal column–medial lemniscal and anterolateral systems are highlighted by the sensory symptoms that follow a hemisection of the spinal cord. Tactile discrimination and limb proprioception, which are relayed by the dorsal columns, are lost in the ipsilateral arm and leg, whereas pain and temperature sense, which are relayed by the anterolateral system, are lost in the contralateral arm and leg.

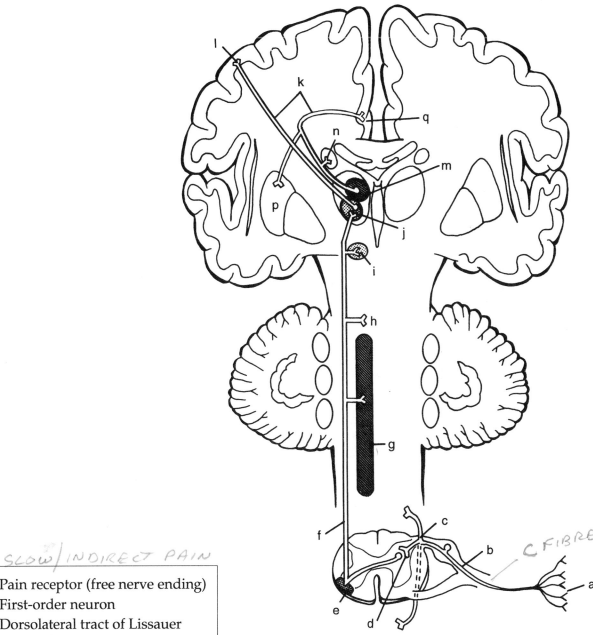

SLOW/INDIRECT PAIN

C FIBRE

a	Pain receptor (free nerve ending)
b	First-order neuron
c	Dorsolateral tract of Lissauer
d	Lamina V
e	Spinothalamic tract
f	Second-order neuron (paleospinothalamic tract)
g	Reticular formation
h	Periaqueductal gray
i	Superior colliculus
j	Posterior nucleus
k	Third-order neuron
l	Parietal lobe (outside S-I)
m	Intralaminar nucleus
n	Caudate nucleus
p	Putamen
q	Limbic cortex

Fig. 11-6

The Somatic Sensory Cortex

The primary somatic sensory cortex (S-I) plays an important role in processing all of the submodalities of the sensory system. It is located in the anterior region of the parietal lobe (postcentral gyrus) and consists of four anatomically distinct areas (1, 2, 3a, and 3b of Brodmann; Fig. 11-7). Area 1 receives input from rapidly adapting receptors in the skin, area 2 receives input from pressure and joint position receptors in deep tissue, area 3a receives input from muscle spindles, and area 3b receives input from rapidly and slowly adapting receptors in the skin. Each area contains a unique topographic representation. The input to the primary sensory cortex comes from the opposite side of the body and projects via the ventral posterior tier of the thalamus. Output from the primary motor cortex goes to several places: the contralateral primary sensory cortex; the contralateral dorsal column–medial lemniscal system and ipsilateral ventral posterior lateral thalamus to control input; the ipsilateral motor cortex and basal ganglia for motor control; and the secondary somatic sensory cortex.

The secondary somatic sensory cortex (S-II) is located on the superior bank of the lateral sulcus.

Tertiary somatic sensory cortex is located in the insula (at the base of the lateral fissure) and posterior parietal lobe. These regions integrate somatic sensory information with other information (e.g., visual and memory) to form complex abstract perceptions.

Clinical Aspects

Lesions of the parietal lobe, seen commonly in cerebrovascular accidents involving the middle cerebral artery, affect the primary, secondary, and tertiary somatic sensory cortices. Cortical lesions alter all somatic sensory information from the opposite side of the body. Unlike thalamic lesions that produce severe disruption of all sensory modalities, cortical lesions produce only minimal disruption of primitive sensory discrimination involving pain, temperature, touch, and vibration but severe deficits in joint position sense, two-point discrimination, touch localization, and the ability to recognize objects placed in the hand (astereognosis). This pattern of loss is referred to as cortical sensory deficit. Primitive perception is formed in the thalamus and thus remains after cortical lesion; localization and discrimination are performed by the cortex and are thus severely diminished after cortical lesion.

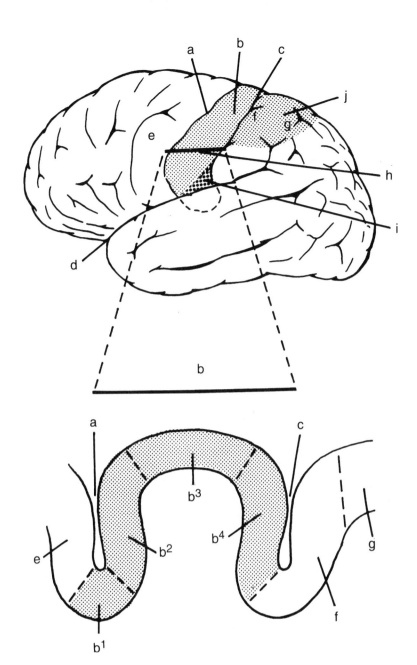

Fig. 11-7

a	Central sulcus
b	Postcentral gyrus
b^1	Area 3a
b^2	Area 3b
b^3	Area 1
b^4	Area 2
c	Postcentral sulcus
d	Lateral sulcus
e	Area 4
f	Area 5
g	Area 7
h	Primary sensory cortex (S-I)
i	Secondary sensory cortex (S-II)
j	Posterior parietal lobe

12 Visual System

Overview

Vision is the dominant sensory modality in humans. For a visual image to be formed, the eyes must be positioned so that photoreceptors, located in the retina, can sense the electromagnetic waves of light reflected from the visual target. Before an image is formed on the retina, the light is refracted by the cornea and lens. The optical properties of the lens invert and reverse the projection of the visual field onto the retina such that the retinal image is upside down and backwards. Once the receptors are activated, they project the retinal image to the occipital cortex, where a visual image of the outside world is perceived. Like other sensory systems, the visual system is crossed such that information from the left visual field is projected to the right visual cortex. It is interesting that in all major sensory and motor systems the central projection pathways are crossed and cortical representations of the external world (visual field, sensory and motor homunculi) are all inverted.

The retina and its associated neurons are actually extensions of the central nervous system. Embryonically, the visual apparatus is derived from an evagination of the diencephalon that migrates to the periphery. The peripheral structure develops into the eyeball, which maintains its innervation during migration. Once in place and fully developed, the visual system extends from the frontal to the occipital poles, forming the horizontal axis of the brain.

Oculomotor System

The extraocular muscles direct the eyes to specific targets in the visual field so that images of these objects fall on corresponding points in both retinas. Eye movement is accomplished by the contraction of extraocular muscles that are under the command of oculomotor, trochlear, and abducens cranial nerves (III, IV, and VI, respectively). Movement of both eyes in the same direction simultaneously (conjugate movement) requires the extraocular muscles to work in synergistic pairs. For example, horizontal lateral gaze to the left requires the simultaneous contraction of the left lateral rectus and right medial rectus muscles (and relaxation of their antagonists; Fig. 12-1). Such complex coordination is achieved through the integration of cortical, brain stem, and cranial nerve control centers.

Four basic types of eye movements are recognized. Each is activated by an independent control system involving different regions of the brain. The first type of movement, fast saccadic eye movement, is used during voluntary searching movements and occurs on command from the frontal eye field (area 8 of Broadmann; Fig. 12-2). This movement occurs so quickly that

the visual image is suppressed movement. Activation of area 8 causes movement of the eyes in the opposite direction. The speed of the saccade is coded in the frequency of neuronal discharge and the extent of movement excursion is coded in discharge duration. The second type of movement, slow pursuit or tracking movement, occurs while following a moving object (e.g., watching a moving car). This type of movement is controlled from areas 18 and 19 of the visual cortex. The third type of movement, vestibuloocular reflex eye movement, serves to maintain the fixation of the eyes on a visual target while the head is moving. It requires coordination of the skeletal muscles moving the head with the extraocular muscles moving the eyes and is performed by the vestibular system through the medial longitudinal fasciculus. The fourth type of movement, vergence eye movement, is used while maintaining fixation on a visual target as it moves from the far visual field to the near visual field. Vergence (convergence) movements are controlled from cortical areas 19 and 22.

All four types of eye movements are used by a departing tourist standing on the ship's deck during the bon voyage party. The tourist scans the dock for a familiar face using saccadic eye movements from face to face. The streamer thrown to well-wishers is tracked using smooth pursuit movement. If an offshore wind blows the streamer back onto the deck below, vergence eye movements combine with smooth pursuit movements to track the streamer from far to near visual fields. Throughout the party, the tourist uses vestibuloocular reflex movements to compensate for head movements caused by the rocking of the ship.

The actual movement of the eyeball within the orbit is accomplished by the six extraocular muscles. Their anatomy and physiology are summarized in Fig. 12-1 and Table 12-1. The integrity of the oculomotor system may be checked by asking the client to move the eyes in the six cardinal directions of gaze (horizontal to the right and left, up and down with eyes right and then left). Horizontal movements test the medial and lateral recti muscles. When an individual looks to the right, the right eye is elevated and depressed by the superior and inferior recti muscles, respectively, and the left eye is elevated and depressed by the inferior and superior oblique muscles, respectively. It should be noted that the recti muscles act in the direction indicated by their names, but the obliques do not. Because of the point of attachment and pulley system used by the oblique muscles, the superior oblique muscle is able to rotate the eye downward and the inferior oblique muscle rotates the eye upward (see Fig. 12-1).

The extraocular system positions the eyes so that the desired image falls onto the preferred portion of the retina. The sensory receptors (rods and cones) then pick

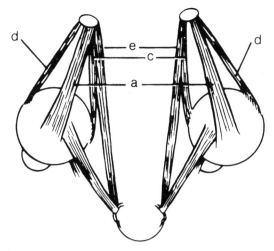

Fig. 12-1

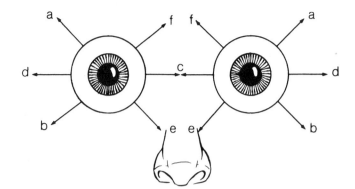

(a–f)	*Extraocular muscles*
a	Superior rectus
b	Inferior rectus
c	Medial rectus
d	Lateral rectus
e	Superior oblique
f	Inferior oblique
g	Frontal eye field
h	Occipitoparietal eye field

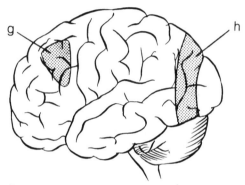

Fig. 12-2

Table 12-1   Muscles and Eye Movements

Muscle	Nerve	Direction of Eye Movement	Signs of Dysfunction
Medial rectus	III	Medial	Eye is deviated down and out with complete paralysis of CN III (usually associated with ptosis and mydriasis)
Superior rectus		Up and out	
Inferior rectus		Down and out	
Inferior oblique		Up and in	
Superior oblique	IV	Down and in	Limitation of downward gaze when eye is looking medially, extorsion of eye
Lateral rectus	VI	Lateral	Eye is deviated medially

up the image and project it to the primary visual cortex. The receptor apparatus consists of both nonneural and neural structures. Almost the entire eyeball is composed of nonneural structures that collect and focus light waves onto the neural retina. The neural structures that make up the retina initiate sensation and the transmission of nerve impulses. Visual perception is complete when the impulses have been received, integrated, and interpreted by the visual cortex. The visual system, from the eye to the visual cortex, forms the horizontal axis of the brain (Fig. 12-3).

Nonneural Peripheral Structures

The nonneural structures of the eye include the cornea, sclera, anterior chamber, iris, lens, and vitreous humor (Fig. 12-4A). The cornea is a transparent membrane that covers the anterior chamber and joins with the white sclera. The sclera provides the supportive covering to which the extraocular muscles attach. The iris is a circular diaphragm with a central aperture, the pupil, through which light projects to the posterior wall. The iris provides the color of the eyes, which depends on the amount of pigment present. The ciliary body supports the lens, a transparent, elastic structure that changes its shape to focus light waves from varying distances onto the retina. The vitreous humor is a transparent gelatinous material that provides support to the inside of the eyeball and separates the lens and retina. The choroid lies behind the retina and prevents the light from scattering after it passes through the retina.

These nonneural structures, along with the extraocular muscles, refract and focus the light rays on the neural structures in the back of the eye. The iris opens and closes in response to varying intensities of light, thereby controlling the illumination of the retina. The lens focuses the image onto the surface of the retina. The lens also inverts the image so that the top of the visual field falls on the bottom of the retina and the left portion of the visual field falls on the right portion of the retina (Figs. 12-3 and 12-5).

Neural Peripheral Structures

During embryonic development, when the optic vesicle migrated to the periphery, its neural innervation grew along with it so as to maintain contact. Neural structures include the retina, optic nerve, and optic tract. The retina developed and grew in such a way that the photoreceptors (rods and cones) face inward toward the back of the eye and are covered by several layers of cells (Fig. 12-4B). Both rods and cones, which were named for their shapes, synapse with first-order sensory neurons (bipolar cells). Bipolar cells, in turn, synapse with second-order ganglion cells, which lie adjacent to the vitreous humor. Horizontal cells and amacrine cells are interneurons that affect the neural processing in the retina by modulating the activity of bipolar and ganglion cells. Light rays must first penetrate layers of ganglion cells, interneurons, and bipolar cells before reaching the photoreceptors.

Ganglion cells are the only output cell from the retina. They collect from throughout the retina before exiting the eye by piercing the sclera at the lamina cribrosa. Beyond the eye, ganglion cells form the optic nerve. The inside of the lamina cribrosa is covered by the optic disk, the only nonneural portion of the retina. In the area up to the optic disk, all retinal cells are unmyelinated and exhibit slow, decremental conduction of nerve impulses. From the optic disk on, fibers become myelinated and exhibit fast, nondecremental conduction.

Throughout most of the retina, there is extensive convergence. There are estimated to be more than 100 million rods and 7 million cones and only 1 million ganglion cells. Thus, individual ganglion cells have large receptive fields on the retina derived from the input of many rods and cones. However, at the posterior pole of the retina, ganglion cells are modified to form a depression, the macula lutea. At the apex of the macula is the fovea centralis. Although cones are present throughout the retina, their density increases abruptly at the macula and they are the only receptors present in the fovea. In the fovea there is a one-to-one relationship between cones and ganglion cells, and this unitary relationship produces the increased acuity of the fovea and makes it the most sensitive region of the retina.

The retina has a consistent structure and density with a higher percentage of rods in the periphery. Rods are the photoreceptors that are sensitive to low-intensity illumination. They are roughly 20 times more numerous than cones and are responsible for black-white (scotopic) vision. These receptors function maximally in

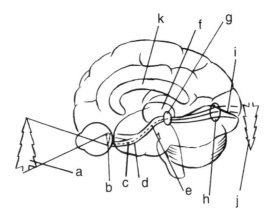

Fig. 12-3

a	Visual target
b	Retinal image
c	Optic nerve
d	Optic chiasm
e	Optic tract
f	Thalamus
g	Lateral geniculate body
h	Optic radiation fibers
i	Primary visual cortex (calcarine sulcus, area 17)
j	Cortical image
k	Corpus callosum

the evening or at night when illumination is beneath the minimum required for cones to function. Rods contain the photopigment rhodopsin, a vitamin A derivative, which is activated on exposure to low-level illumination. Photons of light trapped by the photopigment activate second messengers that are involved in the neural signal of the rod. This is the only light-dependent phase of visual excitation. As the nerve impulse passes from the retina to the optic disk, the receptor potential is transformed into a generator potential and a burst of impulses in the ganglion cell of the optic nerve. Until the transformation at the optic disk, all electrical activity inside the eye was via local potentials. After its breakdown by light, rhodopsin is resynthesized, a process that takes a few minutes. An example of the interval between depletion and resynthesis, when the rods have insufficient rhodopsin with which to function, is the temporary blindness that results from leaving a sunny afternoon and entering a movie theater. During that time, the illumination is too low for cones to function and rods must await the resynthesis of rhodopsin. The resulting blindness is due to the lack of functioning photoreceptors and is relieved when the rods have resynthesized adequate levels of their photopigment. Rods are of particular importance in detecting movement, and light from the blue end of the spectrum (wavelengths of approximately 450 µm) is the most effective in activating rhodopsin.

Cones are the receptors that provide color (photopic) vision. They have a higher threshold and require more illumination than rods. Reflecting their role in color vision, cones differ in their sensitivity to particular wavelengths. Three basic types of cone cells have been identified, each of which is sensitive to one primary color: blue, green, or red. The cones have been named B, G, and R for their color sensitivity. Each of the three types of cone cells contains a different pigment that maximizes absorption of light in a different part of the visual spectrum. Photopigments are named for the type of cone within which they are found: B cones contain B pigment, G cones contain G pigment, and R cones contain R pigment. This specialization underlies trivariant color vision (color vision based on three types of receptors, each most sensitive to one primary color).

Individual cones do not transmit information about the wavelength of a light stimulus. When a cone absorbs a photon, the electrical response it generates is always the same, whatever the wavelength of the photon. Although the wavelength of the photon does not shape the response of the cone, the number of photons absorbed by a cone does vary with wavelength and the more photons absorbed, the higher the discharge frequency. To detect color, the brain compares the responses of the three types of cones, each of which is most sensitive to a different part of the visible spectrum. This trivariancy of color vision explains why any color can be produced by appropriate combinations of blue, green, and red.

The color perceived depends on the wavelengths of light that penetrate the eye. Objects achieve their color from the wavelengths that they reflect and make available in the environment. All wavelengths not reflected are absorbed by the object. The presence of all wavelengths in the visual spectrum stimulates all three types of cones equally, and the color white is perceived. When an object absorbs all wavelengths of light, no cones are stimulated and the color black is perceived. All other colors represent the different combinations of cones stimulated by the light reflected by the object.

Within the visual system, color information is processed by a specialized subsystem. The segregation of color information from information about form and movement starts in the retina. Information about color is then processed by the parvocellular-blob system that includes the lateral geniculate body and area V4 of the primary visual cortex.

In addition to encoding the form, color, and location of an object in the visual field, rods and cones are susceptible to receptor adaptation. This global phenomenon of receptor physiology, if allowed to occur in the visual system, would produce the perception of stable objects as disappearing from the fixed visual field. This unacceptable, unrealistic situation is avoided by the eyes normally making involuntary, continuous, small, rapid, irregular oscillations (microsaccades) when gaze is fixed on an object. Therefore, adaptation is avoided because no retinal image remains immobile.

Central Visual Pathway

The central visual pathway includes the optic nerve, optic chiasm, optic tract, and lateral geniculate body of the diencephalon; the pretectal area of the midbrain (superior colliculus); and the optic radiations and visual cortex of the telencephalon (Fig. 12-5).

Diencephalic Structures

The optic nerve consists of the axons of ganglion cells whose cell bodies are located in the retina. These axons become myelinated as they leave the back of the eye. The optic nerve exits the orbit via the optic foramen to enter the cranium. Although classified as the second cranial nerve, the optic nerve functions as a nerve tract similar to those found in the spinal cord. Like other tracts, the optic nerve consists of second-order sensory neurons that are myelinated by oligodendrocytes rather than Schwann cells. Thus, demyelination diseases that affect the central nervous system, such as multiple sclerosis, produce similar effects in the optic nerve, thereby producing the visual symptoms of the disease.

Once inside the cranium, the optic nerve from each eye unites to form the optic chiasm. Within the chiasm a partial crossing occurs; the fibers from the nasal hemiretina (the half of the retina closest to the nose) cross to the opposite side, while fibers from the temporal hemiretina (the half of the retina closest to the temporal bone) remain uncrossed. From the chiasm back fibers project as the optic tract. In binocular vision, objects

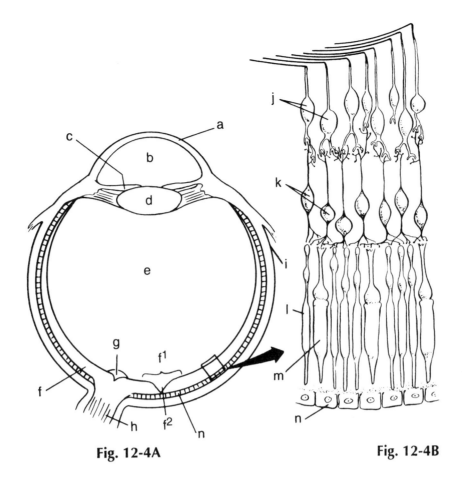

Fig. 12-4A

Fig. 12-4B

a	Cornea
b	Anterior chamber
c	Iris
d	Lens
e	Vitreous humor
f	Retina
f^1	Macula lutea
f^2	Fovea centralis
g	Optic disk
h	Optic nerve
i	Sclera
j	Bipolar cells
k	Ganglion cells
l	Rods
m	Cones
n	Choroid

from the left visual field are projected onto the temporal portion of the right retina and the nasal portion of the left retina (Fig. 12-5). Similarly, objects from the right visual field are projected onto the temporal portion of the left retina and the nasal portion of the right retina. In the chiasm, retinal images are combined because the nasal portion of each retina crosses. The left optic tract then transmits the image from the entire right visual field and the right optic tract transmits the image from the entire left visual field. By this organization, the left visual cortex receives a complete image from the right visual field and the right visual cortex receives a complete image from the left visual field.

After leaving the optic chiasm, each optic tract projects to the thalamus of the same side. Eighty percent of optic tract fibers synapse in the lateral geniculate body and the remaining 20 percent descend into the midbrain to the pretectal area.

Mesencephalic Structures

A small percentage of fibers from the optic tract project beyond the thalamus and establish synaptic connections in and around the superior colliculus. Fibers from this pretectal area project to the cerebral cortex in an area of the frontal eye field (area 8 of Brodmann). This pathway participates in cortically mediated visual reflexes.

Telencephalic Structures

From the lateral geniculate body, fibers project to the primary visual cortex on the banks of the calcarine sulcus (area 17 of Brodmann). These fibers, the optic radiation, reach the cortex by way of the internal capsule. Visual images are received from the environment in such a way that they are inverted on the retina. The retinal image is then projected straight back to the visual cortex, where the image remains inverted (see Figs. 12-3 and 12-5). The primary visual cortex thus has a topographic organization. The association areas of the visual cortex (areas 18 and 19 of Brodmann) lie lateral to the primary visual cortex on either side.

The abstraction of visual information becomes more complex as one moves from area 17 to 18 to 19. Point-to-point visual perception occurs in area 17. Areas 18 and 19 perform higher and higher levels of abstraction on visual information. For example, the convergence of individual points of light is necessary to form the perception of a line and thereby define the shape of an object. The line must then be compared with the background if movement is to be perceived. These progressively higher levels of abstraction necessitate the integration of more and more pieces of information. Within the visual cortex, many cells from area 17 converge onto a single cell in area 18 and many cells from area 18 converge onto a single cell in area 19. Thus, the activity of cells in area 19 underlies the perception of

an object moving through the visual field at a given speed and direction.

Clinical Aspects

Disorders of the visual system produce specific, readily identifiable visual defects, depending on the part of the system that is damaged (Fig. 12-6). Knowledge of these defects permits precise localization of most lesions. Because the visual system forms the horizontal axis of the brain, such information also provides an indirect means for testing brain structures that lie along the same axis.

Disorders of the nonneural structures of the eye are the most common and primarily involve difficulties in focusing. Nearsightedness (myopia), farsightedness (hyperopia), and diseases of the cornea or lens, such as cataracts and glaucoma, all involve focusing problems in the affected eye. (Any of these disorders can occur in both eyes simultaneously and to varying degrees of severity). Disorders of the retina also involve monocular visual loss. The most common retinal disorders include detached retina, retinal degeneration, and vascular disease. Lesions involving part of a single optic nerve may produce a deficit or hole in the visual field (scotoma). If the entire optic nerve is sectioned, all vision originating from that eye is lost (ipsilateral monocular blindness). The most common lesion of the optic chiasm involves the crossing fibers from the nasal portion of the retina, which produces a loss of both temporal visual fields (bitemporal hemianopia). Rarely, the uncrossing fibers from the temporal portions of the retina will be damaged in the chiasm, producing a loss of both nasal visual fields (binasal hemianopia). Lesions of the optic tract, lateral geniculate body, or optic radiations on one side produce homonymous defects in the opposite visual field. For example, a lesion that destroys any of these structures on the left side produces a homonymous hemianopia in the right visual field of both eyes. Lesions involving the visual cortex produce a homonymous hemianopia in the contralateral visual field. However, if the lesion is incomplete, there is often macular sparing or a persistence of the macular or central region of the visual field.

Color blindness can be caused by genetic defects in photopigments or by retinal disease. The most common causes of color blindness are recessive mutations of the X chromosome involving the production of photopigment, not the receptors or the neural circuitry. The genes for the green and red pigments are located on the X chromosome. Approximately two percent of men are green blind and one percent are red blind. Only rarely does genetic mutation affect B type photopigment. Acquired forms of color blindness involve diseases of the outer layers of the retina that usually produce blue blindness (tritanopia) and diseases of the inner layers of the optic nerve that usually produce green and red blindness (protanopia).

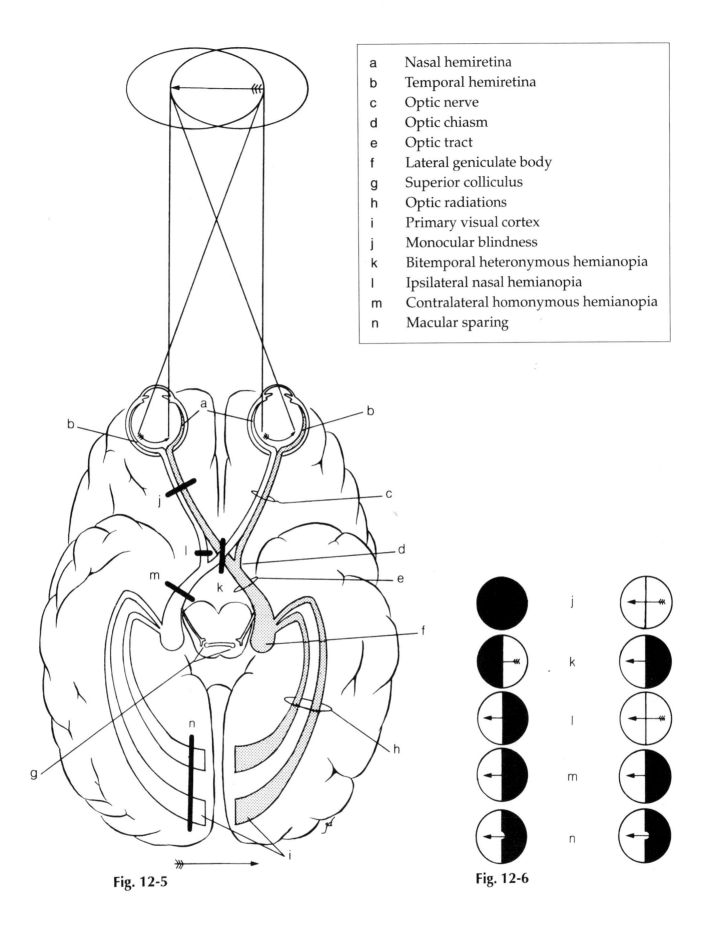

a	Nasal hemiretina	
b	Temporal hemiretina	
c	Optic nerve	
d	Optic chiasm	
e	Optic tract	
f	Lateral geniculate body	
g	Superior colliculus	
h	Optic radiations	
i	Primary visual cortex	
j	Monocular blindness	
k	Bitemporal heteronymous hemianopia	
l	Ipsilateral nasal hemianopia	
m	Contralateral homonymous hemianopia	
n	Macular sparing	

Fig. 12-5

Fig. 12-6

13 Auditory System

Overview

The auditory system subserves hearing, that is, the ability to sense and perceive sound. The system extends from the ear into the brain stem and up to the cortex of the temporal lobe. It transduces mechanical energy (sound waves) into electrochemical nerve impulses. Auditory information is used for communication and to help activate the reticular core of the brain.

Sound is produced when air molecules are compressed and expanded. Sound travels in sinusoidal waves as air molecules compress and expand against adjacent air molecules. The frequency of the waves, measured in hertz (Hz), determines the pitch of the sound. The loudness of the sound, measured in decibels (dB), is determined by wave amplitude. The human ear can detect sound frequencies from about 20 to 20,000 Hz and loudness from about 1 to 120 dB.

Receptor Anatomy and Physiology

The auditory apparatus consists of three components: the outer, middle, and inner ear (Fig. 13-1A). The outer ear consists of the auricle (external ear) and external auditory meatus (ear canal). The middle ear consists of the tympanic membrane (eardrum) and ossicles: the malleus, incus, and stapes (Fig. 13-1B). The inner ear is located in the labyrinth of the temporal bone and contains the cochlea, vestibule, and semicircular canals. The cochlea houses the receptors of sound while the vestibule and semicircular canals house the receptors of head movement.

Sound waves traveling in the environment are picked up by the auricle, channeled down the external auditory meatus, and focused onto the tympanic membrane. The arrival of sound waves causes the thin, flexible tympanic membrane to begin moving, which in turn sets the ossicles into motion. The tympanic membrane and ossicles are not merely the passive recipients of sound waves but are an independently controlled lever system. They exhibit variable stiffness, regulated by the tensor tympani and stapedius muscles. Muscular contraction alters bony alignment, which results in an increased dampening or in less sound being transferred from the outer to the inner ear. Muscular relaxation results in amplified sound transfer. The foot of the stapes rests on the oval window of the cochlea and when the ossicles move the flexible oval window is set in motion. Movement of the oval window causes pressure waves in the perilymph fluid inside the cochlea. The fluid waves cause motion in the hair cells located inside the cochlea and the movement of hair cells produces an increase in the discharge frequency of first-order neurons.

The cochlea consists of three parallel chambers coiled two and a half times into the shape of a helix (snail shell). The two outer chambers, scala vestibuli and scala tympani, are continuous at the apex (helicotrema) and filled with perilymph fluid (Fig. 13-1B). The middle chamber, scala media (cochlear duct), is filled with endolymph fluid and contains the auditory receptor, the organ of Corti (Fig. 13-1C). The scala vestibuli is separated from the scala media by the vestibular (Reissner's) membrane, and the scala tympani is separated from the scala media by the basilar membrane. At the base of the cochlea, the scala vestibuli ends in the oval window and the scala tympani ends in the round window. The fluid waves that start at the oval window travel up the scala vestibuli, across the helicotrema, and down the scala tympani, and are damped at the flexible membrane that covers the round window. As the wave travels down the scala tympani, it sets the basilar membrane and organ of Corti in motion.

The organ of Corti contains two types of hair cells that extend from the basilar membrane to the tectorial membrane (Fig. 13-1D). The hair cells, inner and outer, are named for their position with respect to the tunnel of Corti. The tallest hairs (stereocilia) of outer hair cells are embedded into the inferior surface of the tectorial membrane while hairs from the inner hair cells merely rest in a groove on the undersurface of the tectorial membrane. The hairs act as mechanoreceptors. Movement of the basilar membrane causes the hair to bend, thereby opening ion channels at its base. Movement of ions through the open channels causes the hair cell to depolarize. Hair cell depolarization, in turn, causes the release of neurotransmitter into the synapse, producing an increased discharge frequency in the first-order neuron that wraps around its base.

The following represents the entire stimulus process that produces hearing. Sound waves are collected in the auricle and funneled down the external auditory meatus onto the tympanic membrane, and set the ossicles into motion. Movement of the ossicles establishes waves inside the cochlea that cause movement of the basilar membrane and bending of the attached hair cells. Movement of the hair cells causes deformation of the nerve ending wrapped around the base of the hair cell and results in nerve impulses being generated and conducted in the cochlear nerve.

The structure of the auditory receptor from the auricle to the hair cell in the organ of Corti consists of nonneural tissue. Neural tissue is not encountered until the first-order sensory neurons (bipolar cells) that wrap around the base of the hairs. These neurons exit the cochlea at the apex and form the cochlear portion of the eighth cranial nerve.

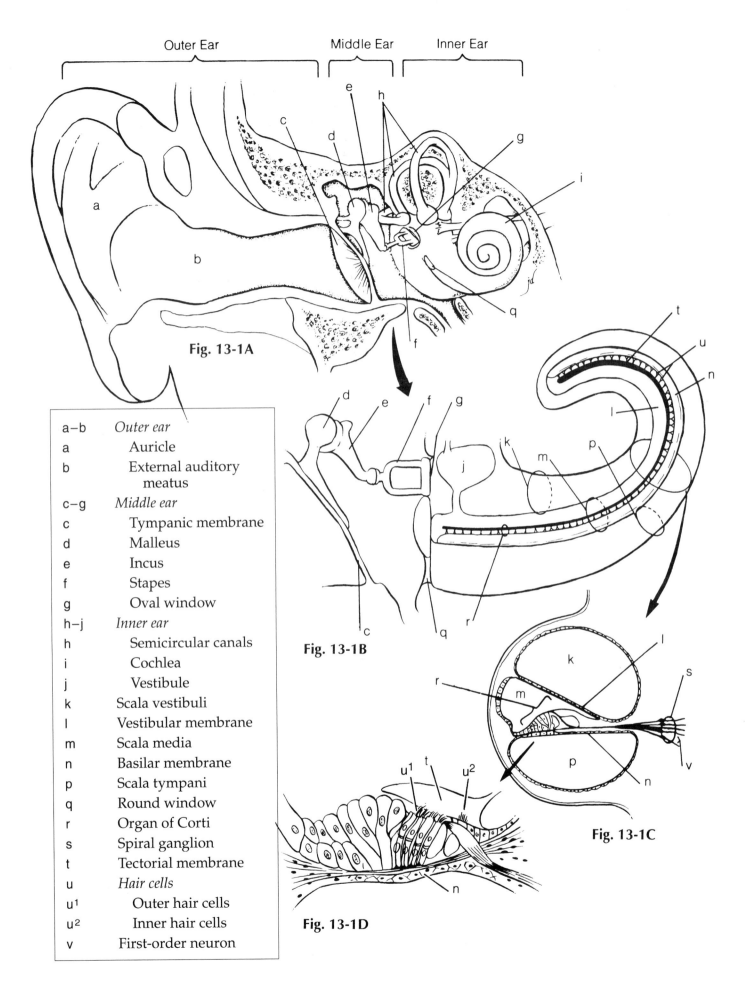

Outer Ear | Middle Ear | Inner Ear

Fig. 13-1A

a–b	*Outer ear*
a	Auricle
b	External auditory meatus
c–g	*Middle ear*
c	Tympanic membrane
d	Malleus
e	Incus
f	Stapes
g	Oval window
h–j	*Inner ear*
h	Semicircular canals
i	Cochlea
j	Vestibule
k	Scala vestibuli
l	Vestibular membrane
m	Scala media
n	Basilar membrane
p	Scala tympani
q	Round window
r	Organ of Corti
s	Spiral ganglion
t	Tectorial membrane
u	*Hair cells*
u¹	Outer hair cells
u²	Inner hair cells
v	First-order neuron

Fig. 13-1B

Fig. 13-1C

Fig. 13-1D

Central Pathway

Auditory information is delivered from the receptors into the central nervous system (CNS) via the eighth cranial nerve, which has two divisions, vestibular and cochlear. Each division is so distinct in its function and anatomical connections that it could be considered as a separate cranial nerve. The vestibular division is considered in Chap. 14.

A small percentage of the central auditory pathway contains a direct, three-neuron projection system from the hair cells in the cochlea to the primary auditory cortex in the temporal lobe. The majority of the central pathway is a bilateral projection system that contains multiple interneurons that ascend through the brain stem and midbrain.

The cell bodies of all first-order neurons are located in the spiral ganglion (Fig. 13-2). Axons project into the brain stem at the junction of the medulla and pons. Each axon bifurcates and establishes synaptic connections in both the dorsal and ventral cochlear nuclei. In the direct pathway, the cell bodies of second-order neurons are located in the dorsal cochlear nucleus. Axons of second-order neurons project dorsal to the inferior cerebellar peduncle in the dorsal acoustic striae, cross the midline, and ascend uninterrupted to the medial geniculate body of the thalamus via the lateral lemniscus. From here, third-order neurons project via the internal capsule to the primary auditory cortex located in the superior temporal gyrus of Heschl (areas 41 and 42) and the secondary auditory cortex, which surrounds the primary auditory cortex (area 22).

Differences in the indirect pathway begin after first-order neurons have synapsed in the cochlear nuclei. Three projections, dorsal, intermediate, and ventral acoustic striae, arise from the cochlear nuclei to relay the information centrally and rostrally. Both the dorsal and intermediate striae are crossed projections and ascend in the lateral lemniscus. The dorsal acoustic striae arise from the dorsal cochlear nucleus and are part of the direct pathway. The other two striae arise from the ventral cochlear nucleus. The intermediate acoustic striae take a course similar to that of the dorsal striae, but, after crossing the midline and ascending in the lateral lemniscus, terminate on neurons in the inferior colliculus. Neurons in the inferior colliculus project to the medial geniculate body, which, in turn, projects to the primary auditory cortex. The ventral acoustic striae provide the bilateral projections of the central acoustic pathway. These fibers pass ventral to the inferior cerebellar peduncle and terminate in the nuclei of the trapezoid body and superior olivary nuclei, bilaterally. These nuclei project fibers into the ipsilateral and contralateral lateral lemniscus. Fibers in the lateral lemniscus ascend through the brain stem to terminate in the inferior colliculus and the nucleus of the lateral lemniscus. From the inferior colliculus, fibers ascend to the medial geniculate body and on to the primary auditory cortex, ipsilaterally and contralaterally.

The central auditory pathway also contains descending neurons that terminate at all levels of the system. It is believed that these efferent fibers act as feedback loops to modulate afferent input. Olivocochlear fibers terminate either directly on hair cells in the organ of Corti, or on afferent fibers of the spiral ganglion. The efferent fibers in the auditory system may be responsible for selective auditory attention and changing the threshold of the hair cells as protection from loud noises.

Auditory Perception

Auditory information is analyzed for three primary psychophysical factors: tone, loudness, and localization. The basilar membrane extends the length of the cochlea, becoming wider and more pliable as it ascends. Because of this variable stiffness, the highest tones (high frequency and short waves) are perceived or "heard" when the base of the membrane experiences maximal displacement, and the lowest tones (low frequency and long waves) are "heard" when the apex of the membrane experiences maximal displacement. This tonotopic localization of the basilar membrane formed the basis for the spatial theory of tone discrimination (resonance theory). According to this theory, the basilar membrane was considered a string resonator, like the strings of a harp, with a specific location on the membrane vibrating for each tone. However, it has been demonstrated that the entire basilar membrane vibrates in response to pressure waves. The frequency theory of tone discrimination was based on the thesis that individual auditory nerves are tuned to respond to some particular sound frequency, called its "best" frequency. The currently held duplex theory combines elements of both the resonance and frequency theories. In order to discriminate high frequencies, a spatial code must be used, whereas for lower middle-range frequencies both spatial and frequency codes are used. The vibrating stapes sets up traveling waves in the perilymph and basilar membrane. For each tone, the wave height of the vibrating basilar membrane increases to a maximum and then drops off rapidly. Each site of maximal displacement along the membrane corresponds to a specific frequency of sound wave (tonotopic organization). The sites of lesser disturbance along the membrane have, as yet, undetermined functional roles that may be associated with some of the qualities of the sound, such as richness. Also, differences in the electromechanical properties of hair cells along the basilar membrane may play a role in tone discrimination.

Loudness or intensity discrimination depends on the amplitude of the vibration in the basilar membrane. At each location along the membrane, a larger displacement will be perceived as a louder intensity of that pitch. Detecting the location from which a sound emanates is achieved by comparing the time and intensity of the sound as it arrives at the two ears. The inferior

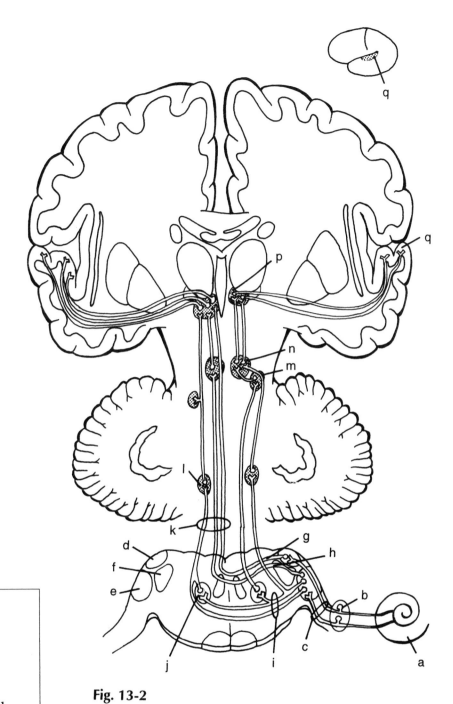

Fig. 13-2

a	Cochlea
b	Spiral ganglion
c	Cochlear division of VIII
d	Dorsal cochlear nucleus
e	Ventral cochlear nucleus
f	Inferior cerebellar peduncle
g	Dorsal acoustic striae
h	Intermediate acoustic striae
i	Ventral acoustic striae
j	Nucleus of the trapezoid body
k	Lateral lemniscus
l	Superior olivary nucleus
m	Nuclei of the lateral lemniscus
n	Inferior colliculus
p	Medial geniculate body
q	Primary auditory cortex

colliculi seem to be central in determining sound localization. Sound originating directly in front, behind, or on top of a person is extremely difficult to locate because the sound reaches each ear at the same time with the same intensity. That is why, in attempting to locate a sound, the head is usually turned so that one ear faces the sound, creating a difference in the time and intensity when the sound reaches either ear.

Clinical Aspects

Lesions of the peripheral auditory system, including the first-order neuron, produce complaints of tinnitus (buzzing or ringing) or deafness (loss of hearing). Unilateral lesions of the central auditory system seldom produce significant alterations in hearing. Unilateral hearing loss usually indicates disease in the ipsilateral ear, eighth cranial nerve, or its nuclei. Conduction deafness is due to disease of the external or middle ear that prevents sound waves from reaching the cochlea. Sensorineural deafness is due to disease of the cochlea or auditory nerve and its nuclei. These conditions can be distinguished by audiometric testing.

Clinical evaluation of the auditory nerve and brain stem centers below the inferior colliculus is performed using the auditory brain stem response (ABR) and acoustic reflex.

14 Vestibular System

Overview

The function of the vestibular system is to signal changes in head position or motion. The reference used to detect these changes is the pull of gravity. Vestibular input is integrated with visual and proprioceptive information to provide the basis on which the central nervous system maintains equilibrium and develops a sense of spatial awareness.

The vestibular system originates from sensory receptors located in each ear, projects directly into the brain stem, bifurcates, and extends as far rostral as the cerebral cortex and as far caudal as the spinal cord. The vestibular system provides information concerning gravity, rotation, and acceleration. This information is extremely important in developing a subjective sensation of motion and regulating the orientation of the body in space. In particular, the motor system relies on vestibular input to control posture, balance, and equilibrium as well as to coordinate movements of the head and eyes. While the vestibular system does project to the cerebral cortex, it is primarily a subcortical system with powerful influence on the spinal cord, affecting muscle tone and reflex activity.

Vestibular Receptors

The receptors of the vestibular system are hair cells in the saccule, utricle, and ampullae of the semicircular canals, all of which are located in the bony labyrinth of the inner ear (Fig. 14-1A, B). The saccule, utricle, and ampullae are chambers filled with endolymph fluid and house the receptor organs. The saccule and utricle each contain a macula and the three ampullae, one at the end of each semicircular canal, each contain a crista. The maculae and cristae contain hair cells that respond to mechanical deformation and are moved by the endolymph that fills the three chambers. Nerve impulses from these receptors are transmitted directly to the vestibular nuclei located in the ipsilateral pons and medulla via the vestibular portion of the vestibulocochlear nerve (CN VIII).

The hair cells in the saccule and utricle respond to changes in head position by sensing changes in the linear direction in which gravity is pulling the hair cells.

The saccule and utricle contain a receptor called the macula, which consists of a base of epithelial support cells from which hair cells project into a gelatinous substance covering the macula (Fig. 14-1C). At the top of each hair cell, inside the gelatin mass, is a small, round, calcified otolith. When the head is tilted, the pull of gravity on the otoliths distorts the hair cells and initiates generator potentials in the vestibular nerve. The macula in the saccule is oriented vertically and responds best to up and down movement while the macula in the utricle is oriented horizontally and responds best to forward/backward or side-to-side movement.

The three semicircular canals respond to rotation or angular acceleration in the three planes of space. The canals are placed at right angles to one another so that each canal monitors movement in a separate plane of space. Each semicircular canal contains a receptor similar to the macula called a crista. The crista is located in the ampulla at the base of each canal (Fig. 14-1D). Rotation of the head causes movement of the endolymph within the semicircular canals, distorting the hair cells of the crista and thus initiating generator potentials in the vestibular nerve. Each hair cell in the crista contains one thick fiber (kinocilium) and 75 to 100 thin fibers (stereocilia). The kinocilium provides a physiological reference for distinguishing the direction of motion. When the hair cell bends in the direction of the kinocilium, the first-order neuron depolarizes. When the hair cell bends away from the kinocilia, the first-order neuron hyperpolarizes. Thus, the receptors are able to signal the direction of rotation.

In general, the vestibular receptors provide information about linear and angular motion of the head. Information about linear motion comes from the saccule and utricle and is most useful in determining the static position of the head in space with reference to the vertical pull of gravity. Information about angular motion comes from the semicircular canals and is most useful in detecting movement. Once the central nervous system knows the position of the head in space and its state of motion, it must then integrate other sources of information (notably proprioception and vision) to determine the relation of the rest of the body to the head.

Central Pathways

The vestibular system and its central pathways constitute one of the most widely dispersed special sensory systems. The cell bodies of first-order neurons are located in the vestibular (Scarpa's) ganglion, which is situated within the internal auditory meatus (Fig. 14-2). Distal axons synapse at the base of hair cells in the saccule, utricle, and ampullae. Proximal axons project directly to the superior, inferior, medial, and lateral vestibular nuclei via the vestibular portion of the eighth cranial nerve. The lateral vestibular nucleus receives input primarily from the macula of the utricle. Second-order neurons from the lateral vestibular nucleus both ascend and descend. Ascending fibers join the medial longitudinal fasciculus (MLF) while descending fibers form the lateral vestibulospinal tract. The medial and superior vestibular nuclei receive input primarily from the cristae of the semicircular canals. Second-order

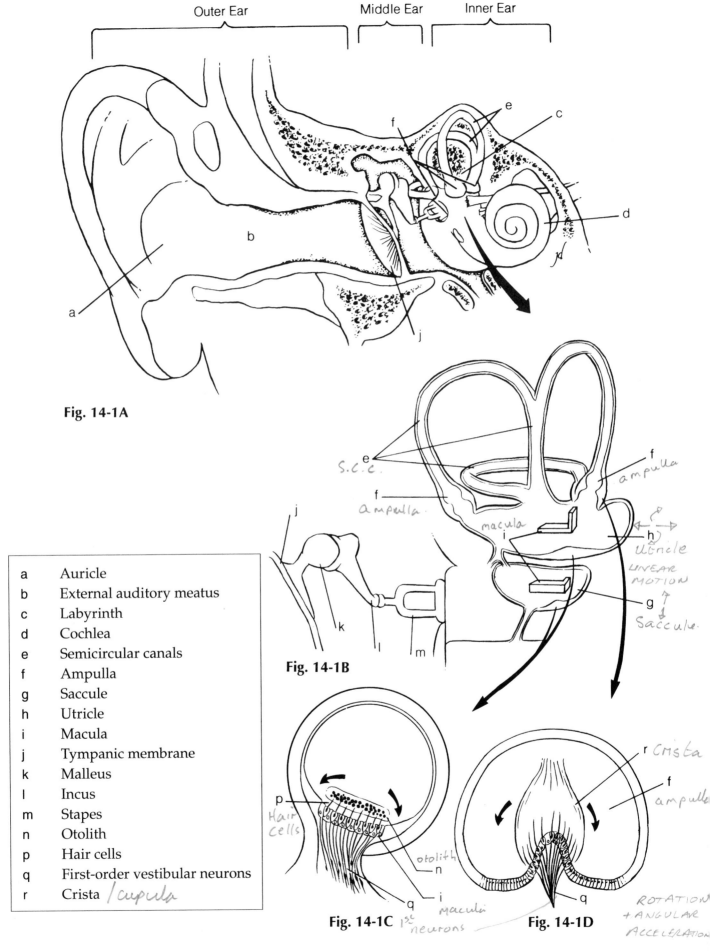

Outer Ear   Middle Ear   Inner Ear

e
c
f
b
d
a
j

Fig. 14-1A

a	Auricle
b	External auditory meatus
c	Labyrinth
d	Cochlea
e	Semicircular canals
f	Ampulla
g	Saccule
h	Utricle
i	Macula
j	Tympanic membrane
k	Malleus
l	Incus
m	Stapes
n	Otolith
p	Hair cells
q	First-order vestibular neurons
r	Crista / cupula

S.C.C.
e
f
ampulla
f
ampulla
macula
i
h
Utricle
LINEAR MOTION
g
Saccule

j
k
l
m

Fig. 14-1B

p
Hair Cells
otolith
n
q
i
macula
1st neurons

r Crista
f
ampulla
q

ROTATION + ANGULAR ACCELERATION

Fig. 14-1C   **Fig. 14-1D**

neurons from these nuclei join both the ascending and descending portions of the medial longitudinal fasciculus. The inferior vestibular nucleus receives input from all three receptors: saccule, utricle, and semicircular canals. The inferior vestibular nucleus projects into the ascending medial longitudinal fasciculus.

Some first-order neurons do not synapse in the vestibular nuclei but project directly to the cortex in the flocculonodular lobe of the ipsilateral cerebellum via the inferior cerebellar peduncle. The flocculonodular lobe, in turn, projects back to the inferior and lateral vestibular nuclei bilaterally via the fastigial nucleus.

Ascending Projections from the Vestibular Nuclei

From their location at the base of the fourth ventricle, the vestibular nuclei project second-order neurons to all levels of the brain stem as well as to specific locations in the cerebellum, thalamus, and cerebral cortex. In addition to the second-order neurons that form reciprocal connections with the cerebellum, most ascending vestibular projections travel via the medial longitudinal fasciculus and regulate vestibuloocular reflexes. The vestibular system is critical in the reflexive control of conjugate eye movement in response to head movement. Second-order vestibular neurons synapse with the cranial nerves (oculomotor, trochlear, and abducens) that determine the position of the eyes.

Second-order vestibular neurons also provide an important source of input to the reticular formation. Although the vestibular system is primarily subcortical, a small percentage of second-order neurons project to the ventral posterior inferior nucleus of the thalamus. Vestibular input has been recorded in the cerebral cortex of the parietal (face region of the postcentral gyrus, areas 2 and 5) and temporal lobe (adjacent to the primary auditory cortex, areas 41 and 42). Presumably, cortical projections came by way of third-order neurons from the thalamus.

Descending Projections from the Vestibular Nuclei: Vestibulospinal Tracts

Two major projections into the spinal cord arise from the vestibular nuclei: the lateral and medial vestibulospinal tracts. The lateral vestibulospinal tract arises from the lateral vestibular tract, and extends uncrossed to the lumbosacral region of the spinal cord. The medial vestibulospinal tract originates from the medial vestibular nucleus, and extends bilaterally through the cervical region of the spinal cord as part of the descending medial longitudinal fasciculus. Both vestibulospinal tracts terminate almost exclusively on interneurons in laminae VII and VIII, which in turn synapse with alpha and gamma lower motor neurons in lamina IX. Both tracts strongly facilitate motor neurons innervating antigravity muscles. These effects support stretch reflex mechanisms in extensor muscles used to support the body against gravity and maintain an upright posture.

Clinical Aspects

Disruption of vestibular function produces disequilibrium, vertigo (the hallucination of rotary movement), and nystagmus (rapid involuntary movement of the eyes in a horizontal, vertical, or rotary direction). The vestibular system balances input from either ear and integrates it with input from other sensory systems to produce the perception of motion. When bilateral vestibular input does not balance because of a malfunction in one or both ears, disequilibrium in the form of dizziness, light-headedness, or wooziness is experienced. Vertigo is usually indicative of a lesion involving the peripheral receptors, vestibular nerve, or brain stem. Vertigo is often accompanied by nausea, vomiting, ataxia, and nystagmus. Nystagmus may be a normal response to visual stimuli or occur as a result of a disturbance in the vestibuloocular system. For this reason, it is indicative of a lesion involving the vestibular nerve, vestibular nuclei, vestibulocerebellar pathways, or vestibuloocular projections. Vestibular nystagmus involves a slow eye movement in one direction resulting from abnormal vestibular stimulation and a fast saccadic corrective component that returns the eye to its original position. It is named for the fast portion of the movement. The function of the vestibular system may be tested by using caloric stimulation or oculocephalic reflexes.

Ménière's disease is a vestibular condition characterized by sudden attacks of severe vertigo and nystagmus accompanied by varying degrees of nausea, vomiting, and postural collapse (falling). Often tinnitus or unilateral deafness is present. The condition is thought to be due to edema, with increased pressure in the membranous labyrinth.

Increased vestibular stimulation is both a source of pleasure and pain. The neurophysiology common to most playground and arcade attractions (slides, swings, merry-go-round, Ferris wheel, or roller coaster) is increased vestibular stimulation. Most families include members who thrive on this increased stimulation and at least one member who knows firsthand the direct connections between the vestibular system and the vomit center. The varying degrees of discomfort (dizziness, light-headedness, headache, nausea, or vomiting) associated with repetitive motion (motion sickness) are due to increased vestibular stimulation.

Finally, the abnormal posturing associated with serious brain injury is due to hyperactive brain stem and midbrain pathways. Decerebrate posturing (marked rigidity of the extensor muscles of the trunk and limbs, with adducted and internally rotated shoulders) occurs following massive, bilateral cerebral trauma; anoxic damage; or destructive midbrain lesion (brain stem transection). Normal muscle tone is the product of

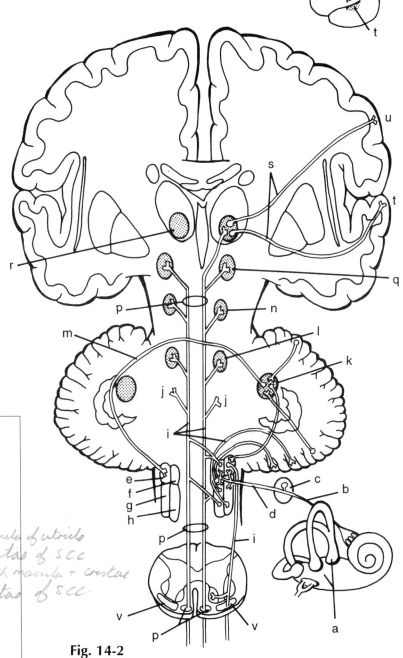

Fig. 14-2

a	Vestibular receptors
b	Vestibular portion of VIII
c	Vestibular ganglion
d	First-order neuron
e–h	*Vestibular nuclei*
e	Lateral *input from macula of utricle*
f	Superior *input from cristae of SCC*
g	Inferior *input from both macula + cristae*
h	Medial *input from cristae of SCC.*
i	Second-order neuron
j	Reticular formation
k	Fastigial nucleus
l	Abducens nucleus (VI)
m	Uncinate fasciculus
n	Trochlear nucleus (IV)
p	Medial longitudinal fasciculus
q	Oculomotor nucleus (III)
r	Ventral posterior inferior nucleus
s	Third-order neuron
t	Temporal lobe adjacent to auditory area
u	Parietal lobe, head region
v	Vestibulospinal tract

a balanced input of excitatory and inhibitory activity from cerebral hemispheres via the descending motor pathways to the level of the lower motor neuron pool. Transection of the brain stem produces excessive activity in the vestibulospinal and reticulospinal tracts by removing the modulating influence from the cerebral hemisphere. Decerebrate rigidity is produced by a marked tonic excitation of gamma motor neurons in the spinal cord. Increased gamma drive increases the discharge frequency of muscle spindle afferents, which reflexively increases the discharge rate of alpha motor neurons to extensor muscles. Decerebrate rigidity is abolished by cutting the vestibulospinal or reticulospinal tracts, which interrupts the hyperactive drive, or by cutting the dorsal roots, which interrupts the hyperactive reflex loop. Decorticate posturing (marked rigidity of the extensor muscles of the trunk and lower extremities accompanied by marked rigidity of the flexor and internal rotator muscles of the upper extremities) occurs following a massive, bilateral lesion above the level of the red nucleus. Transection above the level of the red nucleus "releases" descending pathways from the midbrain and brain stem. Tonic hyperactivity in the rubrospinal tract produces upper-extremity flexor spasticity, and tonic hyperactivity in the vestibulospinal and reticulospinal tracts produces extensor spasticity in the trunk and lower extremities. Lesions large enough to produce decerebrate or decorticate posturing are life threatening, usually accompanied by coma, and predictive of a poor functional outcome following rehabilitation.

15 Gustatory System

Overview

The gustatory (taste) system originates from receptors in the oral cavity, projects directly into the brain stem, and ascends as far as the cerebral cortex in the parietal lobe. Gustatory receptors transduce soluble chemical stimuli into electrical signals that are perceived by the brain as basic taste categories. In conjunction with the olfactory and somatic sensory systems, the gustatory system provides information about the taste of food. This information is used to determine which substances are eaten and, therefore, has obvious survival value.

The word "taste" is generally used synonymously with "flavor," which is a subjective perception based on information from several sensory modalities. Vision and olfaction, along with temperature and tactile senses, play a large part in determining the taste of a substance. Four taste modalities are recognized in humans: salt, sweet, sour, and bitter. Many taste sensations, such as those from numerous spices, fruits, and vegetables, are impossible to describe using the four "elementary taste categories." In fact, an objective schema for classifying all tastes does not exist. The four elementary taste modalities are probably indicative of how little is clearly understood about this complex sensory modality. However, it seems clear that taste is basically a chemically induced sense.

Receptor Anatomy and Physiology

Gustatory receptors are epithelial taste buds that line the papillae of the tongue, palate, and pharynx. Papillae are ridges of tissue that can be readily seen on the edges of the superior surface of the tongue. Taste buds consist of a cup-like configuration of epithelial cells, with tiny hair cells (microvilli) that project into the taste pores lining the sides of the central canal of the papillae (Fig. 15-1). There are three types of papillae in humans: Fungiform papillae are located on the ante-

rior two thirds of the tongue, circumvallate papillae are found on the posterior third of the tongue, and foliate papillae are located on the posterior edge of the tongue. Taste buds found on the palate, epiglottis, and esophagus are not located in papillae.

Individual taste buds consist of three types of cells: nonneural support cells that provide structure for the receptor; basal cells located at the base of the taste bud that act as transition cells, eventually differentiating to become receptor cells; and between 50 and 150 receptor cells. Taste buds are embedded in the epithelium of the papilla and open to the surface with the taste pore, which is lined with microvilli that extend from the apical surface of each receptor cell. The microvilli are thought to be the sites at which sensory transduction occurs. All substances must be water soluble to activate the receptor; however, the exact mechanism by which the receptor transduces particular chemicals into nerve impulses remains unknown.

The life expectancy of receptor cells is only from three to five days. As individual cells die, they are replaced by maturing basal cells. The replacement process takes approximately 10 days. The rate of replacement slows progressively throughout life such that in the later decades of life, taste acuity or sensitivity of taste is significantly diminished.

Each taste bud contains approximately 50 receptor cells. Different receptor cells apparently have receptors specific for different chemicals, but the mechanisms of the interactions are not well understood. Each taste bud contains several different types of receptor cells and can respond to several stimuli. The combination of receptor types varies from bud to bud. Distinct receptor cells detect four basic taste qualities: sweet, salt, sour, and bitter. These receptors are distributed such that the tip of the tongue is most responsive to sweet stimuli, the anterior lateral margins to salty, the entire lateral margin to sour, and the back of the tongue to bitter (Fig. 15-1).

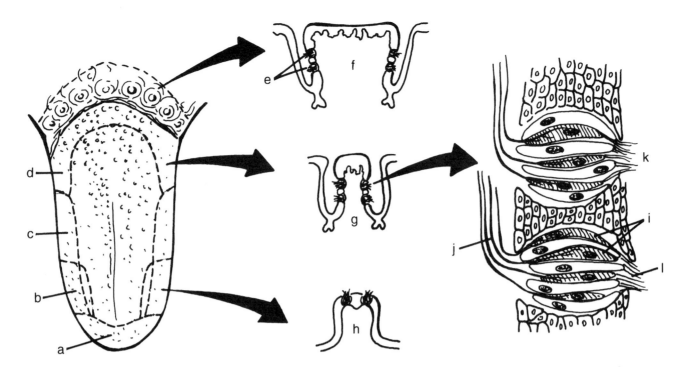

Fig. 15-1

a	Sweet
b	Salty
c	Sour
d	Bitter
e	Taste bud
f	Circumvallate
g	Foliate
h	Fungiform
i	Receptor cells
j	First-order neurons
k	Taste pore
l	Microvilli

Central Pathway

Each receptor cell is innervated at its base by the peripheral process of a first-order neuron. Each peripheral process branches repeatedly, innervating several papillae, several taste buds within each papilla, and several receptor cells within each taste bud. Thus, the information transmitted by a single afferent fiber represents the input from many receptor cells. Receptor cells form chemical synapses with first-order neurons.

Taste buds located in the anterior two thirds of the tongue are innervated by first-order neurons that travel in the chorda tympani branch of the facial nerve (CN VII) with cell bodies located in the geniculate ganglion (Fig. 15-2). Taste buds in the posterior third of the tongue are innervated by first-order neurons that travel in the lingual branch of the glossopharyngeal nerve (CN IX) with cell bodies in the petrosal ganglion. The taste buds on the palate are innervated by first-order neurons that travel in the greater superficial petrosal branch of the facial nerve. The taste buds on the epiglottis and esophagus are innervated by first-order neurons that travel in the superior lingual branch of the vagus nerve (CN X) with cell bodies in the nodose ganglion.

The central process from the first-order neurons in all three cranial nerves terminates in the ipsilateral nucleus solitarius of the medulla. The cell body of second-order neurons comprises the gustatory nucleus located in the rostrolateral portion of the solitary nuclear complex. Second-order neurons from the gustatory nucleus project to the ipsilateral thalamus and terminate in the ventral posteromedial nucleus. In the thalamus, cells serving taste are grouped separately from those related to other sensory modalities of the tongue. Third-order neurons in the gustatory system project from the parvicellular region of the ventral posteromedial nucleus to two regions in the cerebral cortex: the gustatory region in the postcentral gyrus (area 3b of Brodmann) and the face region of the frontal operculum and insula.

Unlike most other sensory systems, the central pathway for gustatory information is not crossed. The somatic sensory information from the tongue projects to the contralateral sensory cortex but gustatory information remains uncrossed.

Clinical Aspects

Loss of taste is called ageusia. Disruption of taste is usually associated with a disorder of one of the cranial nerves that subserves this sense. Because the three nerves serve different regions of the tongue and each region selectively senses different stimuli, individual cranial nerve involvement can be determined by the missing taste category. Since the chorda tympani branch of the facial nerve passes through the middle ear on its way to innervate the anterior two thirds of the tongue, partial ageusia is one possible complication of middle ear disease or surgery. A decrease in the sensitivity of taste often occurs after the age of 40. From birth on, the number of taste buds decreases constantly, but after 40 the drop in taste bud reproduction becomes much steeper. The large number of taste buds present at birth helps account for the greater taste acuity in babies (baby food is only bland to those with fewer buds to taste it). Further, taste buds are not distributed evenly across the tongue. The center of the tongue, with fewer taste buds, is relatively taste-blind. Taste perception contains a heredity factor, so that some individuals are unable to taste certain chemicals, probably due to the lack of specific receptor cells. Preferences and cravings for certain foods change with metabolic conditions, as seen in some pregnant women.

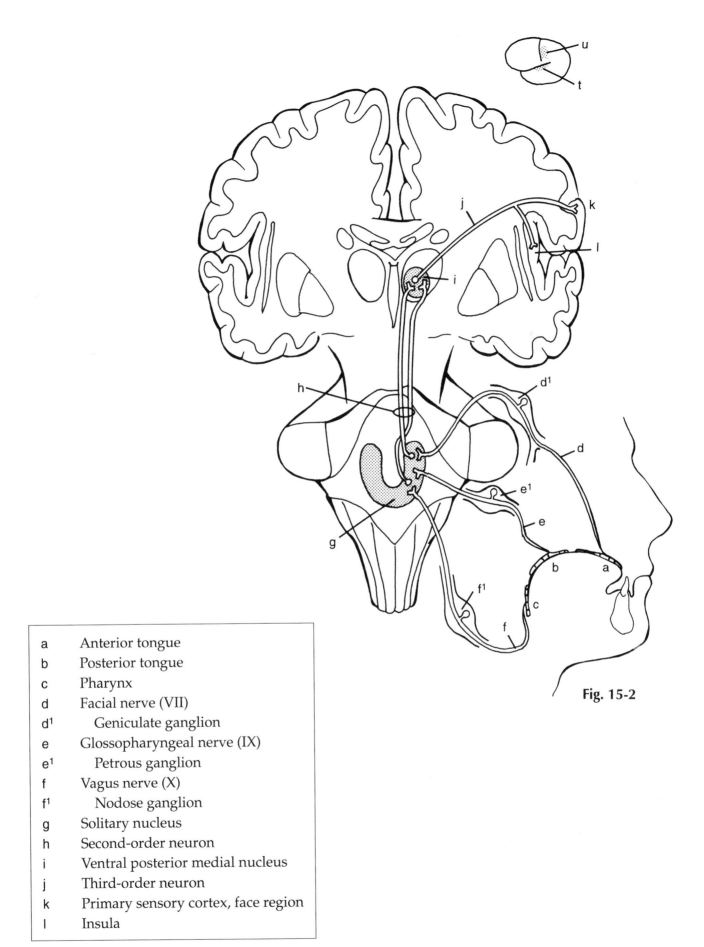

a	Anterior tongue
b	Posterior tongue
c	Pharynx
d	Facial nerve (VII)
d¹	Geniculate ganglion
e	Glossopharyngeal nerve (IX)
e¹	Petrous ganglion
f	Vagus nerve (X)
f¹	Nodose ganglion
g	Solitary nucleus
h	Second-order neuron
i	Ventral posterior medial nucleus
j	Third-order neuron
k	Primary sensory cortex, face region
l	Insula

Fig. 15-2

16 Olfactory System

Overview

The olfactory (smell) system extends from the nose through the skull to the ventral surface of the frontal lobes and back to the cerebral cortex in the temporal lobes. From the temporal lobe, olfactory information projects widely throughout the brain. Olfactory receptors respond to the chemical structure of many substances that are perceived as odors. Olfactory information helps to form the perception of taste.

Receptor Anatomy and Physiology

Olfactory receptors are chemoreceptors located in the mucous membrane that lines the dorsal posterior recess of the nasal cavity, olfactory epithelium (Fig. 16-1A). Receptors are bipolar neurons that have a short peripheral process and a long central process. The short peripheral process extends to the surface of the mucosa, where it terminates as a bulbous olfactory knob. The knob gives rise to several cilia that are embedded in the surface mucosa (Fig. 16-1B). The longer, unmyelinated central process of multiple neurons joins to form bundles of axons and projects through the cribriform plate of the skull as the olfactory nerve (the first cranial nerve). The fibers terminate in the ipsilateral olfactory bulb located on the ventral surface of the frontal lobe.

Olfactory neurons differ from most other neurons in the mammalian nervous system in that they are generated throughout the life of the mature animal. The average life span of an olfactory receptor is approximately 60 days. New receptors develop from precursor basal cells. This constant regeneration is remarkable in that it requires constant synaptogenesis with mitral cells (projection fibers located inside the olfactory bulb).

The exact means by which the chemicals stimulate the receptors remains unknown. It appears that the chemical substance that acts as an olfactory stimulus (odorant) is first absorbed into the mucous layer overlying the receptor. Then, the odorant diffuses to the cilia of the receptor or is presented to the cilia attached to a receptor protein present in the mucosa. A specific protein, known as olfactory binding protein, has been identified. The application of odorants to olfactory receptor sites has two effects. The direct effect is to open sodium channels, depolarizing the receptor and increasing the discharge frequency. The indirect effect is thought to be mediated via second messenger mechanisms.

How discrete chemical compounds are coded for discrimination as different odorants is also poorly understood. Spatial patterns of activation over the surface of the olfactory mucosa play an important part. Although responses to specific odorants occur throughout the olfactory epithelium, different regions of the epithelium show higher sensitivity for individual odorants.

Central Pathway

First-order neurons are bipolar receptor cells that receive support from adjacent nonneural cells. The distal process from bipolar cells extends to the surface of the mucous membrane, where they end as a bushy projection of hair cells. The fine central process forms the unmyelinated olfactory nerve fibers (CN I). Bundles of these fibers pass through the cribriform plate of the ethmoid bone and enter the olfactory bulb. The first synapse occurs within the glomerulus of the olfactory bulb. The incoming olfactory nerve fibers synapse with mitral cells. The lateral olfactory stria consists of fibers that project directly to the primary olfactory cortex (prepyriform cortex and periamygdaloid area) and secondary olfactory cortical area (entorhinal cortex).

Axons from second-order mitral and tufted cells form the olfactory tract, which projects posteriorly along the inferior surface of the frontal lobe (Fig. 16-2). As the olfactory tract reaches the anterior perforated substance, it bifurcates into medial and lateral olfactory striae. The fibers of the medial olfactory stria synapse in the anterior olfactory nucleus with fibers that cross the midline in the anterior commissure and project to the contralateral olfactory bulb. These fibers connect the two olfactory bulbs and modulate the input from the contralateral side. The lateral olfactory stria consists of fibers that project directly to the olfactory cortex, which is located on the medial portion of the ventral surface of the brain and consists of the olfactory tubercle, pyriform cortex, amygdala, and entorhinal cortex.

Input to the olfactory cortex is shared with other portions of the brain via projections through the thalamus and limbic system. The olfactory tubercle and pyriform cortex project to the other olfactory cortical regions and to the orbitofrontal cortex via the dorsomedial nucleus of the thalamus. Together these thalamic and cortical projections are thought to participate in the conscious perception of odors. The cortical nucleus of the amygdala and the entorhinal cortex are portions of the limbic system. These connections are thought to give many odors their strong emotional and visceral qualities. The reflex connections established by these structures produce rapid and forceful behavioral reactions such as the violent nausea that results from putrid odors.

The olfactory system may not be entirely afferent. Following lesion of the olfactory receptors or bulb, some fibers remain intact in the olfactory tract. Although the

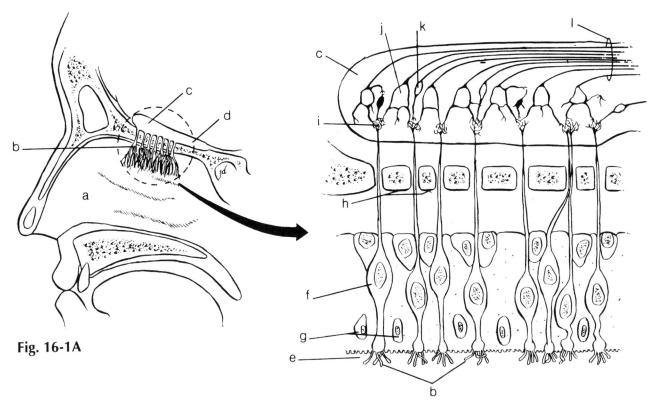

Fig. 16-1A

Fig. 16-1B

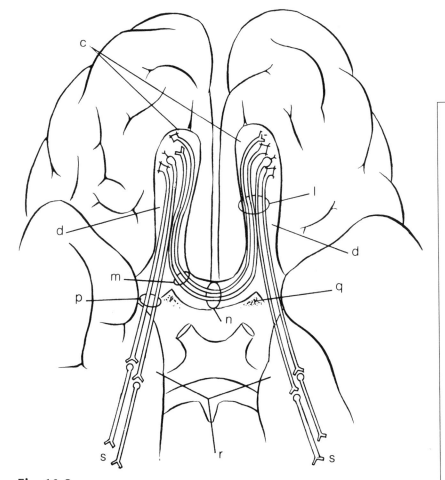

Fig. 16-2

a	Nasal cavity
b	Bipolar cell
c	Olfactory bulb
d	Olfactory stalk
e	Mucous membrane
f	Rods
g	Support cells
h	Cribriform plate
i	Glomerulus
j	Mitral cell
k	Tufted cell
l	Olfactory tract
m	Medial stria
n	Anterior commissure
p	Lateral stria
q	Anterior perforated substance
r	Uncus
s	Olfactory cortex

remaining fibers have not been identified clearly, they may be efferent fibers that control the sensitivity of olfactory receptors.

Clinical Aspects

The olfactory system is of limited clinical importance in humans, although two types of pathology do occur: loss of smell and olfactory hallucinations. Loss of smell (anosmia) may result from infections (including the common cold), trauma, neoplasms, metabolic disorders, and drug ingestion. Diminished sensitivity, if bilaterally symmetrical, is of little clinical importance; however, bilateral imbalance can help to establish the laterality of neurological problems to the side of the diminished sensitivity. Because olfactory and gustatory systems work together, complete anosmia results in an inability to recognize flavors. In addition, the sense of smell may diminish in the later decades of life because the threshold to detect various odors is considerably higher in older people. Finally, a lesion in the region of the medial temporal lobe (uncus) can cause olfactory hallucinations (unusual and disagreeable odors) as part of uncinate epileptic seizures (seizures originating from the uncus).

17 Visceral Nervous System

Overview

Unlike the somatic nervous system, which senses and responds to changes in the external world, the visceral nervous system senses and responds to changes within the environment inside the body. The primary function of the visceral nervous system is to maintain the internal environment within physiological limits (homeostasis). Most visceral regulation is achieved via reflexes at subconscious levels. Components of the visceral nervous system exist at all levels of the neuraxis (forebrain, midbrain, hindbrain, spinal cord, and periphery) and they regulate the function of smooth muscle, cardiac muscle, and glands. To control these effectors, the visceral system uses both neural and humoral (hormones released into the blood) mechanisms.

In addition to neurohumoral differences with the somatic nervous system, the visceral nervous system has two other unique characteristics. First, the effector mechanisms are still capable of functioning in the absence of neural control. For example, cardiac muscle continues to contract rhythmically in the absence of neural innervation. Second, the peripheral level of the visceral nervous system contains ganglia that play an important part in the reflex control of effector function. Visceral ganglia are organized into two systems. The paravertebral ganglia form a chain located immediately adjacent to the vertebral column that extends the entire length of the spinal cord and functions in the sympathetic division of the visceral efferent system. The parasympathetic division of the visceral efferent system contains peripheral ganglia that are located in or around the effector mechanism that they innervate. Table 17-1 compares the somatic and visceral nervous systems.

Visceral Afferent System

The two primary types of visceral receptors, mechanoreceptors and chemoreceptors, are distributed throughout the body. Mechanoreceptors sense pressure, stretch, or tension. Slow-adapting mechanoreceptors sense fullness in the bowel, bladder, and stomach. Fast-adapting mechanoreceptors sense the movement in the lungs and arteries. The second receptor type, chemoreceptors, exist only in the visceral nervous system. As discussed in Chaps. 15 and 16, chemoreceptors sense taste and smell as well as the concentration of hydrogen ions (pH) in the stomach and partial pressure of oxygen and carbon dioxide in the blood. Chemoreceptors located in the hypothalamus and reticular formation respond to the levels of blood sugar and electrolytes. These receptors help the hypothalamus to regulate hunger and thirst.

Visceral afferent fibers are small-diameter, myelinated and unmyelinated axons that exhibit slow conduction velocity. Some first-order visceral afferent fibers project only as far as the peripheral ganglia while others project into the spinal cord and brain stem, and ascend to higher levels of the brain (Fig. 17-1). Two pathways exist for peripheral afferent fibers. They either join with peripheral and spinal nerves to project directly into the spinal cord or they follow blood vessels centrally until reaching a ganglion. The fibers that project to ganglia may either synapse and terminate, pass through the ganglion giving off a collateral synapse, or pass directly through the ganglion and enter the central nervous system (CNS). Visceral afferent fibers that enter the central nervous system have their cell bodies located in the dorsal root ganglia or the sensory portion of a cranial nerve nucleus. To enter the spinal cord, visceral afferent fibers join spinal nerves by projecting through the ganglion and white ramus communicans (communicating branches that are white because they are myelinated) and enter the spinal cord along with the other fibers of the dorsal root. In the brain stem, fibers project directly to cranial nerve nuclei.

The visceral afferent fibers that enter the central nervous system establish multiple synaptic connections at the level of entry. They synapse with both visceral and somatic efferent neurons. Synaptic connections with visceral neurons form the anatomical basis for central visceral reflexes. Synaptic connections with somatic neurons form the basis for associated somatic and visceral behaviors such as the postural collapse that often accompanies severe visceral pain. The convergence of visceral and somatic fibers onto a postsynaptic neuron

Table 17-1   Comparison of Somatic and Visceral Nervous Systems

Component	Somatic	Visceral
Area of concern	External environment	Internal environment
Effector organs	Musculoskeletal system	Smooth muscle, cardiac muscle, glands
Control strategies	Conscious, voluntary	Subconscious, reflexive
Control mechanisms	Neural	Neural and humoral
Effects of denervation	Effectors cease to function	Effectors continue to function
Peripheral apparatus	Spinal and cranial nerves	Prevertebral and paravertebral ganglia

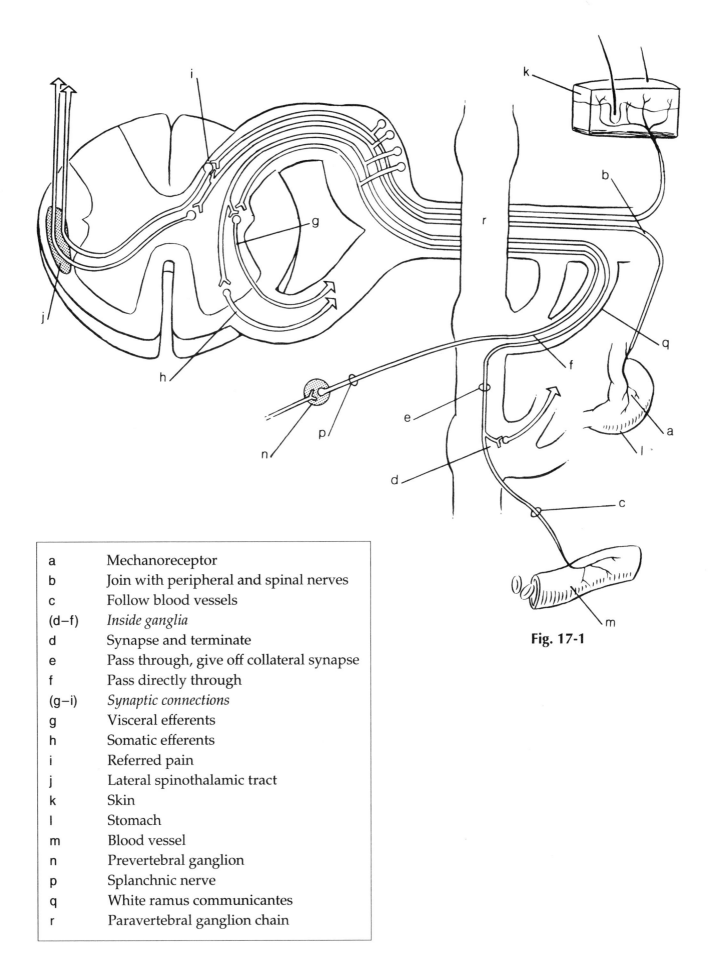

Fig. 17-1

a	Mechanoreceptor
b	Join with peripheral and spinal nerves
c	Follow blood vessels
(d–f)	*Inside ganglia*
d	Synapse and terminate
e	Pass through, give off collateral synapse
f	Pass directly through
(g–i)	*Synaptic connections*
g	Visceral efferents
h	Somatic efferents
i	Referred pain
j	Lateral spinothalamic tract
k	Skin
l	Stomach
m	Blood vessel
n	Prevertebral ganglion
p	Splanchnic nerve
q	White ramus communicantes
r	Paravertebral ganglion chain

forms the anatomical basis of referred pain. Referred pain originates from a deep visceral organ (heart, appendix, etc.) but is "referred" to more superficial areas of the body with the same segmental representation in the spinal cord. Visceral afferent information ascends in the spinal cord and brain stem via the lateral spinothalamic tract and dorsal columns to the reticular formation and then up to the hypothalamus, thalamus, and cerebral cortex.

In spite of cortical projections, the primary destination of visceral afferent activity is the hypothalamus. The hypothalamus is the integrator of visceral information that it receives from the periphery, spinal cord, reticular formation, thalamus, and rhinencephalon. The visceral nervous system contains large numbers of afferent fibers (the vagus nerve contains approximately 80 percent afferent fibers), but conscious perception of visceral sensations is limited to the stomach, bowel, and bladder under normal circumstances. Most visceral function is controlled by subcortical reflexes, which makes diagnosis and localization of visceral dysfunction extremely difficult.

Visceral Efferent System

The visceral nervous system exerts control over smooth muscle, cardiac muscle, and glands via three pathways: sympathetic, parasympathetic, and humoral. Together, the sympathetic and parasympathetic pathways comprise the autonomic nervous system. Both these divisions are two-neuron systems and consist entirely of efferent fibers.

The Sympathetic Division

The sympathetic division has components in the hypothalamus, reticular formation, spinal cord, and periphery (Fig. 17-2). It assumes responsibility for the control of activating types of behavior, such as dilation of the pupil, increased heart rate and respiratory rate, and the shunting of blood to the peripheral musculature, all of which prepare the body to respond to stress. Descending fibers from the hypothalamus and reticular formation are located in the lateral brain stem and spinal cord. The cell bodies of preganglionic sympathetic neurons are located in the lateral horn of the gray matter in the first thoracic through third lumbar segments of the spinal cord (T1–L3). Anatomically, the sympathetic division is referred to as the thoracolumbar division of the autonomic nervous system. Short preganglionic fibers exit the spinal cord via the ventral root and project to the paravertebral ganglia via the white rami communicantes. The white ramus is so colored because preganglionic sympathetic fibers are myelinated.

Once inside the paravertebral ganglion chain (which extends from the first cervical vertebra to the coccyx), preganglionic fibers project in one of three ways (Fig. 17-2). They may synapse immediately with postganglionic fibers, ascend or descend within the ganglion chain before synapsing with postganglionic fibers, or pass through the paravertebral ganglia without synapsing. These direct projecting fibers are myelinated and form the three splanchnic nerves (superior, inferior, and lowest) that synapse in the prevertebral ganglia (ciliac, superior mesencephalic, and inferior mesencephalic). Before synapsing, single preganglionic fibers diverge extensively to form synaptic connection with as many as 10 postganglionic neurons, which distribute sympathetic stimulation widely throughout the body. Long unmyelinated postganglionic fibers exit the ganglia via the gray rami communicantes and provide the sympathetic innervation to effector mechanisms. Postganglionic fibers join with peripheral nerves and project directly to effectors.

Preganglionic sympathetic fibers produce short-lived facilitation of postganglionic neurons by using acetylcholine neurotransmitter substance. Postganglionic fibers produce long-lived, generalized, and specific activation of effector mechanisms by using norepinephrine neurotransmitter substance. Based on the transmitter substance used, most preganglionic fibers are classified as cholinergic and most postganglionic fibers as adrenergic (sweat glands and blood vessels in skeletal muscle are exceptions).

The Parasympathetic Division

The parasympathetic division of the autonomic nervous system arises from the brain stem and sacral segments of the neuraxis and is therefore referred to as the craniosacral division (Fig. 17-2). This division assumes responsibility for regulating restorative types of behavior, including eating, sleeping, and digestion. Stimulation of parasympathetic fibers increases digestion and the absorption of nutrients, drainage of the bowel and bladder, decrease of heart rate and respiratory rate, and shunting of blood to the digestive system from the musculoskeletal system.

Parasympathetic ganglia are located distal to the central nervous system in or near the effector mechanism. Thus, preganglionic fibers are long and postganglionic fibers are short. Both preganglionic and postganglionic fibers of the parasympathetic division produce specific, short-lived effects on postsynaptic membranes by using acetylcholine neurotransmitter substance. The entire parasympathetic division is classified as a cholinergic system.

Long preganglionic fibers from cranial segments exit the central nervous system with efferent fibers from the oculomotor (III), facial (VII), glossopharyngeal (IX), and vagus (X) cranial nerves. Oculomotor, facial, and glossopharyngeal nerves innervate structures in the head and throat. Parasympathetic ganglia in the head region are discrete constellations of neurons, smaller than the head of a pin. The ciliary ganglion is located just behind the eyeball and helps regulate the shape of the lens and diameter of both the lens and the pupil. The sphenopalatine ganglion is found in the lateral wall of the nasal cavity near the nasopharynx and helps to regulate the glands of the eye and nasal and oral cavities. The submandibular ganglion is located

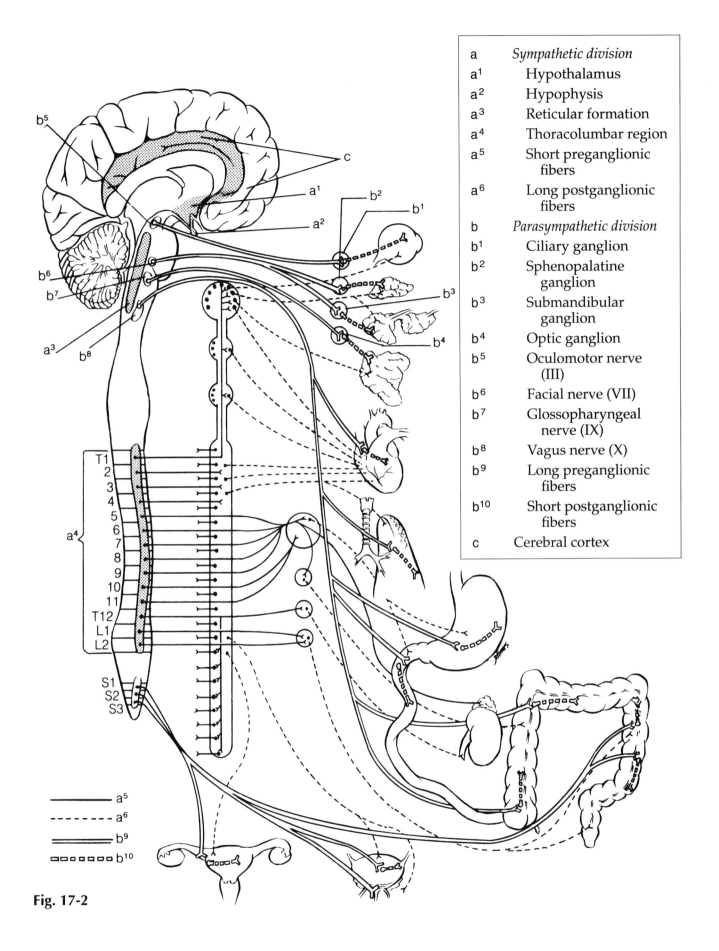

	a	*Sympathetic division*
	a¹	Hypothalamus
	a²	Hypophysis
	a³	Reticular formation
	a⁴	Thoracolumbar region
	a⁵	Short preganglionic fibers
	a⁶	Long postganglionic fibers
	b	*Parasympathetic division*
	b¹	Ciliary ganglion
	b²	Sphenopalatine ganglion
	b³	Submandibular ganglion
	b⁴	Optic ganglion
	b⁵	Oculomotor nerve (III)
	b⁶	Facial nerve (VII)
	b⁷	Glossopharyngeal nerve (IX)
	b⁸	Vagus nerve (X)
	b⁹	Long preganglionic fibers
	b¹⁰	Short postganglionic fibers
	c	Cerebral cortex

Fig. 17-2

inside the jaw and helps to regulate parotid (salivary) glands. The optic ganglion is found just inside the mandible, beneath the temporal bone, and helps regulate sublingual and submaxillary (salivary) glands. The vagus nerve contains approximately 75 percent of all parasympathetic outflow from the cranial region. The vagus nerve provides the parasympathetic innervation to the organs of the thorax and abdomen.

An increase in the parasympathetic activation from the sacral region stimulates digestion and excretion. In the second, third, and fourth sacral regions (S2, S3, S4), the cell bodies of preganglionic fibers are located in the lateral region of the ventral horn. The sacral outflow provides the parasympathetic innervation to the urinary system, lower colon, anal sphincter, and reproductive system. Preganglionic fibers exit the spinal cord via the ventral roots and project in the pelvic nerve to synapse with postganglionic parasympathetic neurons in the pelvic ganglion plexus. Postganglionic parasympathetic neurons innervate the descending colon, bladder, and external genitalia.

Table 17-2 compares the sympathetic and parasympathetic divisions.

The Enteric Division

The enteric division is concerned with control of the gastrointestinal tract, pancreas, and gallbladder. Because these structures contain sensory receptors, afferent neurons, peripheral ganglia, and efferent neurons, their control is sometimes referred to as the enteric nervous system. Although the enteric nervous system is capable of functioning independently, its activity is normally regulated by CNS reflexes. Because of its role in controlling digestion, the enteric division plays a major part in homeostasis. The neurons of the enteric division are arranged in complex interconnecting plexuses of ganglia and nerve fibers located between the layers of muscle and endothelium. Extrinsic innervation of the enteric division is supplied by both the sym-

pathetic and parasympathetic systems. Sympathetic innervation consists primarily of postganglionic fibers from the cervical paravertebral chain. These fibers project to ganglia in the wall of the stomach, small intestine, and colon. Parasympathetic preganglionic fibers project directly to enteric ganglia in the stomach, colon, and rectum through the vagus and pelvic splanchnic nerves. Autonomic innervation, both sympathetic and parasympathetic, provides a second level of control of digestion that is capable of overriding intrinsic enteric control in situations of emergency and stress.

Central Visceral Control

The central control of the visceral nervous system includes three primary areas: the cerebral cortex, hypothalamus, and reticular formation. In the visceral nervous system, cortical centers play a minor role in central control. The two cortical centers, the ventrobasal frontal lobe and the rhinencephalic cortex (medial surface of frontal and temporal lobes), function mainly to integrate somatic and visceral information. Efferent pathways from these areas project directly to the hypothalamus, mamillary bodies, and brain stem reticular formation. There are no direct projections into the spinal cord. Cortical centers coordinate emotional and visceral reactions such as blushing, which is associated with embarrassing situations. The visceral cortex is part of the larger limbic system, which regulates most human emotions and their associated visceral reactions. Limbic and visceral structures are commonly involved in emotional disorders.

The hypothalamus is the major region of central visceral control. All visceral sensory information is projected to the hypothalamus and the hypothalamus has efferent projections to other visceral and limbic areas of the cortex, reticular formation, and spinal cord. Both afferent and efferent visceral pathways are diffusely organized. The hypothalamus has primary responsibility for regulating restorative and preparatory behav-

Table 17-2 Comparison of Sympathetic and Parasympathetic Divisions

Component	Sympathetic	Parasympathetic
CNS segments of origin	Thoracolumbar region of the spinal cord	Craniosacral regions of the spinal cord
Location of ganglia	Paravertebral ganglion chain	On or near effector organ
Preganglionic neuron	Short, myelinated	Long, myelinated
Preganglionic neurotransmitter substance	Acetylcholine	Acetylcholine
Postganglionic neuron	Long, unmyelinated	Short, unmyelinated
Postganglionic neurotransmitter substance	Norepinephrine	Acetylcholine
Divergence ratio	1:10	1:3
Outflow specificity	Can be widespread Can be specific	Specific
Behavior produced with stimulation	"Fight or flight"	Sedentary activities Voiding
Effect on energy stores	Energy mobilization Energy utilization Inhibition of digestion	Energy conservation Energy restoration Stimulation of digestion

ior as well as homeostasis. The anterior hypothalamus controls the posterior hypophysis and parasympathetic system, which regulate restorative types of behavior. The posterior hypothalamus controls the adenohypophysis and sympathetic system, which regulate preparatory types of behavior. The medioventral hypothalamus uses the neurohypophysis to regulate homeostasis.

The reticular formation, the remaining area of importance in the central control of the visceral system, is among the oldest structures in the mammalian brain. It extends from the midbrain through the brain stem and consists of numerous centers that control specific, visceral, life-support functions such as heart and respiratory rates. Reticular centers are not discrete nuclei but, rather, clusters of cells that regulate specific visceral function.

Opposing Mechanisms or Functional Synergy

Most visceral effector organs receive innervation from both postganglionic sympathetic and parasympathetic fibers. Sympathetic neurotransmitter substances (epinephrine and norepinephrine) tend to increase effector function while parasympathetic neurotransmitter substance (acetylcholine) tends to decrease effector function. Both types of efferent fibers are tonically active. Thus, the level of activity of visceral effector organs is determined by the dynamic equilibrium between sympathetic and parasympathetic stimulation. For example, norepinephrine released from postganglionic sympathetic fibers acts on cardiac muscle to increase heart rate and contractility, whereas activation of postganglionic parasympathetic fibers in the vagus nerve causes the release of acetylcholine, which profoundly decreases heart rate and contractility, thereby decreasing cardiac output. Thus, adaptive responses are executed or homeostasis is maintained by varying autonomic drive (sympathetic or parasympathetic) of visceral organs in proportion to external challenges to the system.

Clinical Aspects

High blood pressure, or hypertension, is the most common health problem associated with the cardiovascular system. Hypertension leads to cerebrovascular accidents, heart attacks, and kidney failure, which kill tens of millions of people every year. Hypertension has many causes; however, increased sympathetic drive is one important factor in the development and maintenance of high blood pressure. Sympathetic stimulation increases both cardiac output and peripheral vascular resistance, the two leading determinants of blood pressure. Antihypertensive drugs lower blood pressure by decreasing sympathetic drive. Beta-adrenergic blocking agents reduce the sympathetic drive to the heart, thereby reducing cardiac output. Alpha-adrenergic blocking agents reduce peripheral vascular resistance by interfering with the vasoconstriction produced by the norepinephrine released from sympathetic fibers.

Autonomic dysreflexia or sympathetic hyperreflexia is a specific type of hypertension found in individuals with spinal cord lesions above T7. An abnormal sympathetic response to bladder or bowel distention or painful stimuli in the viscera produces dangerous increases in blood pressure, headache, perspiration, and chills. This response is not self-limiting and is therefore potentially life threatening.

Postural hypotension is a less dangerous though more common blood pressure abnormality. Postural or orthostatic hypotension (low blood pressure) produces light-headedness or fainting after rising from a recumbent or sitting position. The condition results from a failure of the visceral nervous system in sensing and responding adaptively to the change in blood pressure. As the person stands up, gravity pulls the blood into the lower extremities. Unless the tension in the vasculature of the lower extremities is increased proportionately, blood will pool in the legs, perfusion of the brain will drop, and consciousness will be lost. The baroreceptor reflex normally senses and responds automatically to changes in aortic blood pressure in order to maintain blood flow to the brain. The exact cause of postural hypotension, pressure receptors, afferent transmission, CNS integration, peripheral sympathetic or parasympathetic efferents, or effector response to stimulation remains unknown.

Diabetes mellitus produces widespread problems throughout the body, including peripheral neuropathy involving both somatic and visceral neurons. Small-diameter neurons, both myelinated and unmyelinated, are the most vulnerable. The clinical symptoms of autonomic diabetic neuropathy often include cardiovascular control and gastrointestinal motility. The inability to produce and utilize adequate amounts of insulin causes metabolic breakdown and loss of function in the neurons that control these functions.

18 Limbic System

Overview

The components of the limbic system are restricted to the forebrain and midbrain. Unlike other neural control systems, which regulate specific functions such as pain and temperature or movement, the limbic system controls emotions (drive, motivation) and affect. Because of the prominent visceral component in each of these types of behavior, the function of the limbic system is inextricably linked with that of the visceral nervous system, and is therefore sometimes referred to as the "visceral brain." However, functions of the limbic system extend far beyond the visceral nervous system to include the integration of internal and external environments as well as involvement in memory. The limbic system, including its anatomy and physiology, is among the most complex in the entire nervous system and not yet understood fully.

The structures of the limbic system are arranged in a ring or loop located on the medial surface of the cerebral hemisphere and are sometimes classified as the limbic lobe (Fig. 18-1). Limbic structures include the hippocampus, fornix, mamillary bodies, anterior nucleus of thalamus, and cingulate gyrus, as well as regions of the temporal, parietal, and frontal lobes. All sensory systems—auditory, gustatory, optic, tactile, and olfactory—provide highly processed input to the system. The primary output from the limbic system comes via two pathways. The first involves the hypothalamus, brain stem, spinal cord, and somatic motor system. The second involves the hypophysis and makes use of the autonomic and neuroendocrine systems.

Electrical stimulation of limbic structures evokes a variety of sensations as well as somatic motor and autonomic responses. Evoked responses differ depending on the structures stimulated and the nature of stimulation used. Somatic motor responses evoked by limbic stimulation include those associated with acquiring and eating food (sniffing, licking, chewing, swallowing), grooming and goal-seeking, and attack and defense (snarling, clawing, posturing). Autonomic responses evoked by stimulation include changes in heart and respiratory rates, blood pressure, activity of the gastrointestinal tract, and the level of many hormones in the blood. Sensory responses evoked by stimulation include olfactory sensations (unpleasant odors), vertigo, visceral sensations from the abdomen, and pain and pleasure.

The interconnections of the limbic system are highly complex and only partially understood. The most prominent connections can be summarized into three pathways: those within the limbic lobe and associated subcortical structures, those that connect this complex with the diencephalon, and those that con-

nect the diencephalon with the midbrain tegmentum, raphe nuclei, and interpeduncular nucleus.

Pathways Within the Limbic System

Papez's circuit was the first comprehensive and detailed description of the interconnections between limbic structures. The circuit includes projections from the hippocampus via the fornix to the mamillary body, via the mamillothalamic tract to the anterior nucleus of the thalamus, on to the cingulate gyrus, and back to the hippocampus. This closed circuit was viewed as providing the central control of emotion. Since Papez originally described the circuit in 1937, numerous scientists have attempted to specify individual structures and their interconnections that underlie the central control of emotion. As a result of extensive work, a complex anatomical network that interconnects limbic structures has been identified. It is generally agreed, however, that the complex network of limbic structures includes Papez's circuit.

Additional study of the limbic system has identified the hippocampus and amygdaloid nuclear complex as the principal subcortical structures. The hippocampus is interconnected with many regions. Input is provided through projections that come via (1) multineuronal chains from adjacent neocortex of the temporal lobe, which, in turn, receives its input from association areas of the neocortex; (2) the fornix from the septal region; (3) the fornix and hippocampus of the opposite hemisphere (via the commissure of the fornix); and (4) the longitudinal striae from the septal region. This input integrates multidimensional information from many regions of the archicortex.

Output from the hippocampus is transmitted primarily via the fornix. From the fornix, fibers project to the contralateral fornix and hippocampus, septal region, preoptic region, cingulate gyrus, mamillary body, anterior and intralaminar nuclei of the thalamus, lateral hypothalamic nucleus, and rostral central gray matter of the midbrain tegmentum.

The amygdaloid nuclear complex can be divided into two groups of nuclei, the corticomedial and basolateral (Fig. 18-1). The corticomedial group receives its major input from the olfactory bulb. Output from this group projects bilaterally (crossing over in the anterior commissure) via the stria terminalis to the septal region and the preoptic region of the hypothalamus. The basolateral group has many reciprocal connections with the neocortex of the parahippocampal gyrus. These neocortical connections in the temporal lobe lead to other neocortical connections in the frontal lobe and cingulate gyrus. Additional connections of the basolateral group are established through the hippocampus.

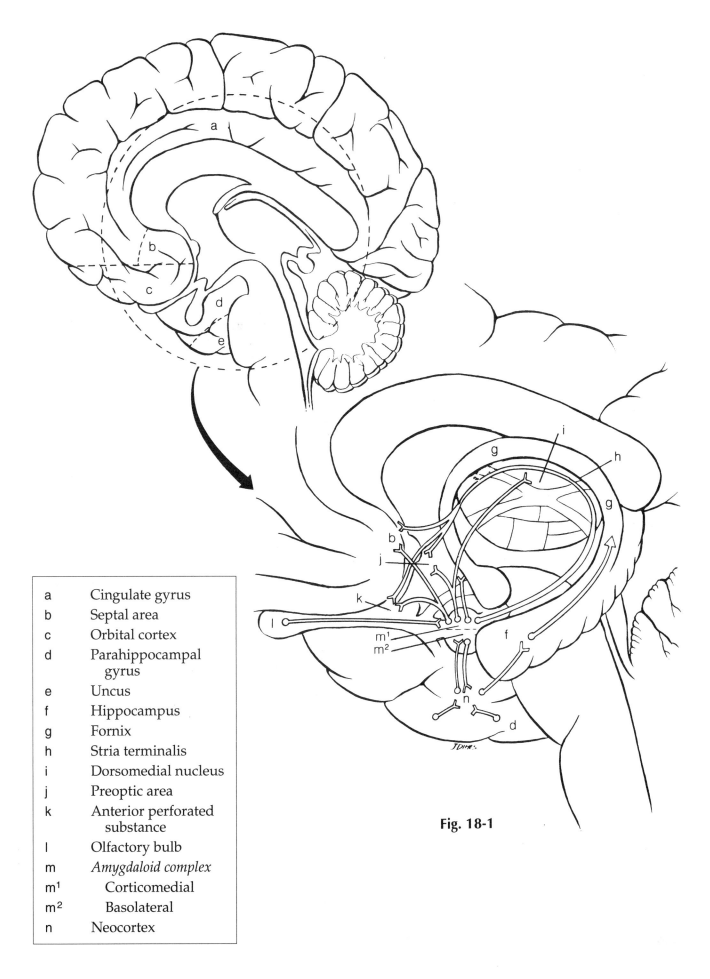

a	Cingulate gyrus
b	Septal area
c	Orbital cortex
d	Parahippocampal gyrus
e	Uncus
f	Hippocampus
g	Fornix
h	Stria terminalis
i	Dorsomedial nucleus
j	Preoptic area
k	Anterior perforated substance
l	Olfactory bulb
m	*Amygdaloid complex*
m¹	Corticomedial
m²	Basolateral
n	Neocortex

Fig. 18-1

The output from the amygdaloid nuclear complex comes via two major pathways: the ventral amygdalofugal fibers and the stria terminalis. Amygdalofugal fibers are larger and project to the lateral, ventral, and preoptic regions of the hypothalamus, dorsomedial nucleus of the thalamus, septal region, and anterior perforated substance.

While the specific functions of the amygdala remain uncertain, experimental and clinical evidence suggest that it is important in linking emotional and motivational responses to external stimuli. It plays a role in learning tasks that require coordination of information from different sensory modalities as well as linking the somatic and visceral components of a response.

The limbic lobe, particularly the hippocampus and amygdala, has been implicated in short-term memory (limited storage of recent events up to a few seconds). Individuals with bilateral lesions of the hippocampus and amygdala retain long-term memory (vast storage of permanent memories) but lose the ability to encode new memories (anterograde amnesia). Similar memory loss is found in thiamine-deficient chronic alcoholics (Korsakoff's syndrome), who, in an effort to disguise this memory loss, will fabricate elaborate answers to questions (confabulate). In Korsakoff's syndrome lesions are also found in the dorsomedial nucleus and pulvinar of the thalamus as well as in the mamillary bodies.

The hippocampus and amygdala are probably not the locale for the storage of the memory trace (engram), but, rather, are involved in the active consolidation necessary to move an item from short-term to long-term memory or retrieve the information from memory. Actual memory storage is thought to involve plastic changes in neurons, including the structure and effectiveness of synaptic connections located in many regions throughout the brain.

Pathways Connecting the Limbic System and Diencephalon

To achieve its profound influence on memory and emotion, the limbic system utilizes extensive connections with the diencephalon (Fig. 18-2A). The hippocampus projects fibers via the fornix to the anterior, intralaminar, and dorsolateral nuclei of the thalamus, lateral hypothalamus, and mamillary body. The amygdala projects fibers via the stria terminalis to the preoptic region of the hypothalamus and the dorsomedial nucleus of the thalamus.

Output from the septal region and the preoptic region of the hypothalamus projects via (1) the stria medullaris thalami bundle to the habenular nucleus of the epithalamus and (2) the medial forebrain bundle to the lateral hypothalamus and tegmentum of the midbrain (Fig. 18-2B). Electrical stimulation of the septal region affects both emotion and visceral functions. Aggressiveness is inhibited or decreased in monkeys and cats by electrical stimulation of the system. Immediately after stimulation ends, dominant or aggressive behavior returns. Also, changes in blood pressure, respiratory rate, and digestion accompany septal stimulation. Stimulation in humans has been shown to produce similar effects.

Pathways Connecting the Diencephalon with the Midbrain

The remaining connection of the limbic system involves pathways that link the diencephalon with the midbrain tegmentum, raphe nuclei, and interpeduncular nucleus (Fig. 18-2B; the raphe nuclei are within the tegmentum and are not depicted). The hypothalamus has three pathways that interconnect with the midbrain. First, the medial forebrain bundle is a complex of reciprocal connections between many hypothalamic nuclei and the midbrain tegmentum. Second, the mamillary body projects to the midbrain tegmentum via the mamillotegmental tract and dorsal longitudinal fasciculus. Third, the habenular nucleus gives rise to the fasciculus retroflexus, which projects to the midbrain tegmentum and interpeduncular nucleus. The interpeduncular nucleus also projects to the midbrain tegmentum.

Electrical stimulation of specific regions within the limbic system of cats, dogs, dolphins, monkeys, apes, and humans has very strong effects on behavior. The stimulation of some sites excites the animal to avoid further stimulation—an expression of negative reinforcement. Such sites have been named pain centers. The stimulation of other sites excites the animal to seek further stimulation—an expression of positive reinforcement. Such sites have been named pleasure centers. Stimulation in either pain or pleasure centers has very strong effects on behavior. Animals will do almost anything to avoid stimulation to pain centers. Conversely, animals with electrodes implanted in pleasure centers will continue to depress a lever that provides self-stimulation rather than eat if hungry or drink if thirsty. In humans, stimulation of a pain center evokes responses of fear or terror and stimulation of a pleasure center evokes responses of "feeling good" or "brightening one's attitude." Pain centers have been located in the midbrain tegmentum and certain areas of the thalamus and hypothalamus. Pleasure centers have been located in the midbrain tegmentum, septal region, cingulate cortex, hippocampus, amygdala, preoptic area of the hypothalamus, anterior nucleus of the thalamus, and medial forebrain bundle. Pain and pleasure centers may be located within a fraction of a millimeter of each other. The medial forebrain bundle and the structures it innervates are effective sites of positive and negative reinforcement.

Clinical Aspects

Before lesions of limbic structures produce symptoms, often they must be bilateral. Bilateral hippocampal lesions lead to memory disorders (anterograde amnesia) by interfering with the neural processing necessary to

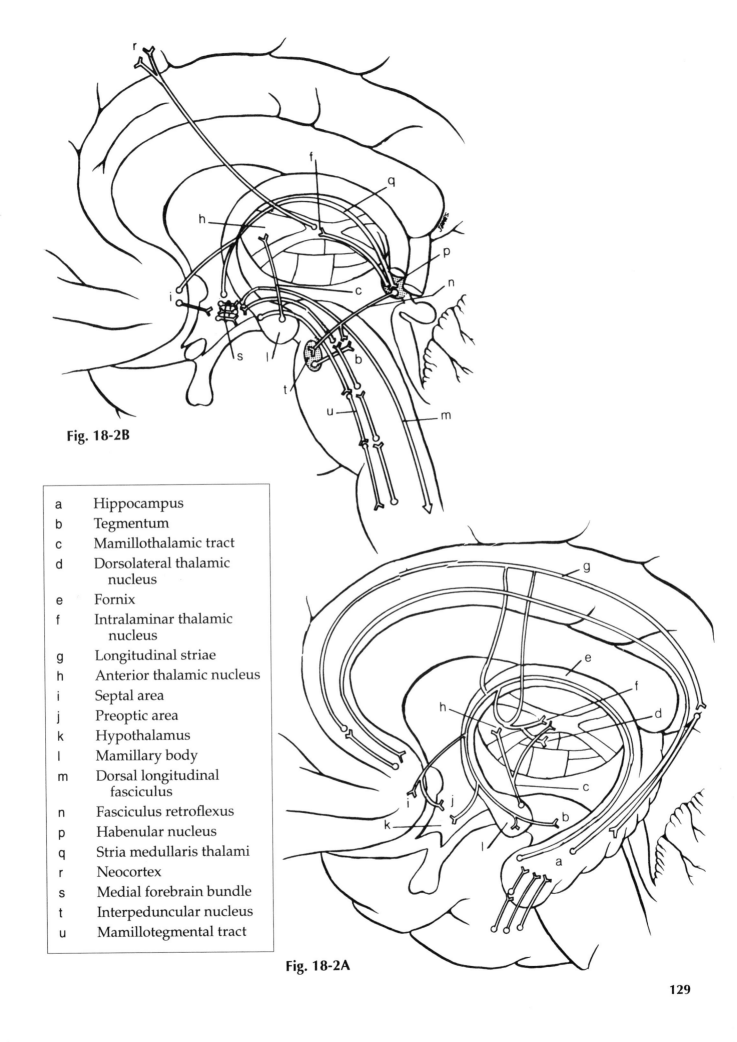

Fig. 18-2B

a	Hippocampus
b	Tegmentum
c	Mamillothalamic tract
d	Dorsolateral thalamic nucleus
e	Fornix
f	Intralaminar thalamic nucleus
g	Longitudinal striae
h	Anterior thalamic nucleus
i	Septal area
j	Preoptic area
k	Hypothalamus
l	Mamillary body
m	Dorsal longitudinal fasciculus
n	Fasciculus retroflexus
p	Habenular nucleus
q	Stria medullaris thalami
r	Neocortex
s	Medial forebrain bundle
t	Interpeduncular nucleus
u	Mamillotegmental tract

Fig. 18-2A

move information from short-term memory to long-term memory. Such lesions have obvious effects on learning. However, once learning has occurred, forgetting seems to occur at a normal rate.

Bilateral lesions of the anterior temporal lobe (including amygdala, anterior temporal cortex, and portions of the hippocampal formation) produce a constellation of behavior known as Klüver-Bucy syndrome. There is an inability to recognize familiar objects, including friends, family, and places, by sight (visual agnosia). Animals with this condition exhibit strong oral tendencies to examine objects repeatedly with their lips and mouth. The object is compulsively touched, smelled, and tasted, presumably in an effort to identify a familiar object that they cannot recall. There is an apparent release from expressing fear, and aggressive animals become docile. There is also a marked absence of emotional response. Some sources indicate that bilateral lesion of only the amygdala will produce the syndrome.

Hyperactivity in the limbic system is also associated with disorders of thought, memory difficulty, and abnormal emotional conditions. Excessive transmission of dopamine in the limbic system is related to schizophrenia.

19 *Cerebral Cortex and Hemispheric Specialization*

Overview

The cerebral cortex is the mantle that covers both cerebral hemispheres and gives them their convoluted superficial appearance. The cortex is generally viewed as the highest functional level of the nervous system and responsible for uniquely human characteristics, such as intricate hand movements, highly developed speech, symbolic thought, personality, conscience, and self-awareness. These qualities are known to depend on the cortex because, if certain areas in the cortex are damaged, these qualities are lost or greatly impaired.

Structural Organization of the Cortex

Structurally, the cerebral cortex contains both horizontal and vertical organization. The horizontal organization consists of six layers made up of two types of neurons (Fig. 19-1). Cortical neurons are classified as either pyramidal or nonpyramidal based on the shape of the cell body. Pyramidal cells have a cell body shaped like a pyramid, with the apex pointing toward the surface of the brain. The apex gives rise to a single apical dendrite that runs toward the surface and intersects intervening layers at right angles. The base of the cell gives rise to several basilar dendrites that course laterally within the layer containing the cell body. Nonpyramidal cells usually have small, round cell bodies with dendrites arising from all aspects of the cell body.

Pyramidal and nonpyramidal cells also differ with respect to their axons. The axon of a pyramidal cell has a main trunk that projects in the white matter to another region of the cortex or to a more distal site within the central nervous system (CNS). In addition to the main trunk, the axon may have collateral branches that terminate near the cell body. In contrast, the axon of the nonpyramidal cell branches profusely and remains in the region near the cell body. Layers with high concentrations of pyramidal cells form the output segment of the cortex while layers with predominantly nonpyramidal cells form the receptive layers for cortical input. This systematic arrangement of pyramidal and nonpyramidal cells produces the horizontal layers in the cortex.

Horizontally, the cortex is divided into six cell layers on the basis of cytoarchitecture (arrangement of cell types, Fig. 19-1). The layers are numbered sequentially from the surface to the myelinated projection fibers that underlie the cortex. Layer 1 (molecular) consists primarily of glial cells and projection fibers running parallel to the surface. Because the projection fibers synapse on the apical dendrites of cells from deeper layers, layer 1 functions to interconnect cortical regions. Layers 2 and 3 (external granular and external

pyramidal, respectively) contain large numbers of pyramidal cells that project to other cortical regions. Layer 4 (internal granular) consists primarily of nonpyramidal cells and forms the primary receptive region for cortical input. Layer 5 (internal pyramidal) contains the largest pyramidal cells and forms the primary output region from the cortex to the rest of the nervous system. Layer 6 (multiform) contains smaller pyramidal cells that project from the cortex to the thalamus.

While the basic six-layer structure remains constant throughout the cortex, the thickness of individual layers varies with the function of the different cortical regions. Based on the changes in microscopic structure, cytoarchitectural maps have been created that divide the surface of the cerebrum into distinct areas. Some areas correspond with recognized function while others do not. The most frequently used cytoarchitectural map was developed by Korbinian Brodmann, a German neurophysiologist, who divided the human cerebral cortex into 52 areas (Fig. 19-2). Functionally distinct areas of the cerebral cortex are often referred to by their Brodmann number designation.

The vertical organization of the cortex consists of columns of cells that respond to a specific type of stimulus from a particular region of the body. The area of the cortex that receives information from the hand contains individual columns specialized for the sensation of touch, pressure, temperature, or pain (see Fig. 19-1). These vertical columns are very important and considered to form the functional units of the cortex. The columns of cells run perpendicular to the layers and together they form the structural and functional organization found throughout the cortex.

The primary function of the cerebral cortex is integration. The anatomical convergence necessary for integration occurs both within columns of cortical cells and between cortical areas. Within individual columns, input is integrated sequentially over time and represented by the ongoing level of activity in that column. Integration between cortical areas occurs as the output from two or more cortical regions converge. Such complex integration is necessary to form holistic perceptions of the way objects feel, taste, smell, look, and relate to the surrounding environment. Transcortical fibers, both those located in layer 1 and projection fibers located in the white matter, provide the pathways for integration of information from distal cortical sites. The exact location in which complex perceptions are formed remains unknown, although association areas of the cortex are probable sites. Neurons that project from one hemisphere to the other are called commissural fibers (corpus callosum, anterior and posterior commissures) and provide for the sharing of information from one hemisphere to the other.

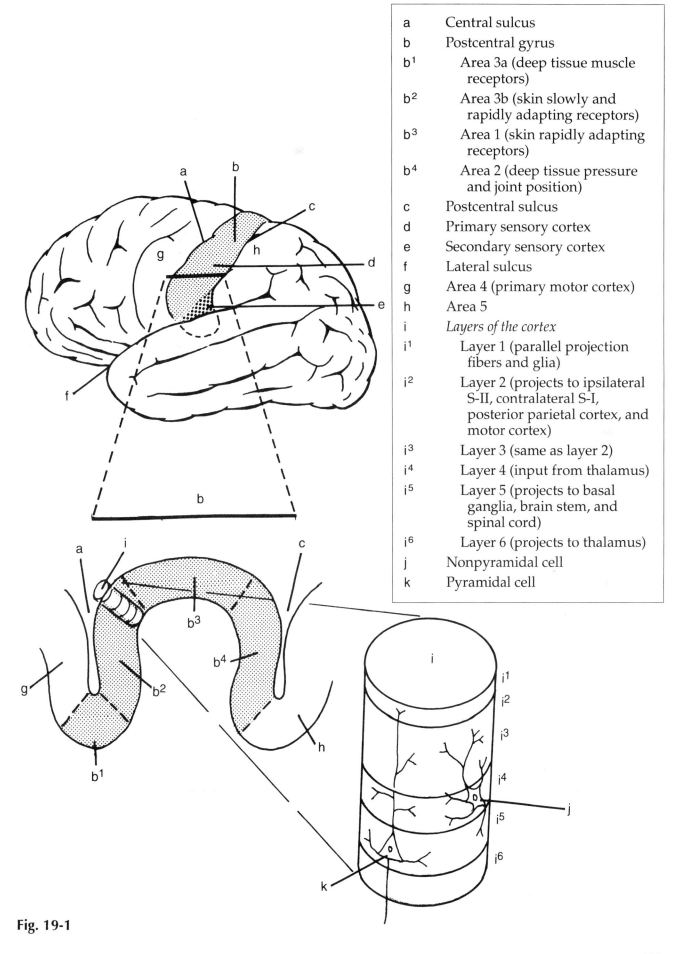

a	Central sulcus
b	Postcentral gyrus
b^1	Area 3a (deep tissue muscle receptors)
b^2	Area 3b (skin slowly and rapidly adapting receptors)
b^3	Area 1 (skin rapidly adapting receptors)
b^4	Area 2 (deep tissue pressure and joint position)
c	Postcentral sulcus
d	Primary sensory cortex
e	Secondary sensory cortex
f	Lateral sulcus
g	Area 4 (primary motor cortex)
h	Area 5
i	*Layers of the cortex*
i^1	Layer 1 (parallel projection fibers and glia)
i^2	Layer 2 (projects to ipsilateral S-II, contralateral S-I, posterior parietal cortex, and motor cortex)
i^3	Layer 3 (same as layer 2)
i^4	Layer 4 (input from thalamus)
i^5	Layer 5 (projects to basal ganglia, brain stem, and spinal cord)
i^6	Layer 6 (projects to thalamus)
j	Nonpyramidal cell
k	Pyramidal cell

Fig. 19-1

Functional Organization of the Cortex

Functionally, the cerebral cortex contains two types of areas: one that is dedicated to specific functional systems and one that is responsible for associating or integrating information from other areas. Cortical regions identified with specific functional systems are referred to as primary, secondary, and tertiary projection areas. Cortical projection areas are often referred to by their Brodmann number designation, for example, primary visual, 17; secondary visual, 18; tertiary visual, 19; primary motor, 4; premotor, 6; frontal eye field, 8; primary somatosensory, 3a, 3b, 2, 1; primary olfactory, 38; primary auditory, 41 and 42; and so forth. Regions of the cortex that are responsible for integrating information from functional systems are referred to as association areas. The majority of the space in each lobe is occupied by association areas. An example of cortical integration is seen when the color, taste, shape, smell, and texture of a spherical citrus fruit are integrated to produce the concept of "an orange."

The cerebral cortex is also somatotopically organized such that the body surface may be represented or mapped on the cortex (see Fig. 11-1). The most widely described examples of this somatotopic arrangement are found in the primary motor cortex (area 4) and primary sensory cortex (areas 3, 1, 2). There are two important aspects about this representation of the body or homunculus. First, the map is distorted such that some body parts have greater representation than others. Second, the homunculus is inverted with the lower extremity represented on the medial aspect of the hemisphere and the head on the lateral aspect adjacent to the lateral fissure. Both the distortion and the inversion have important functional consequences. The body parts with the greatest cortical representation have the most precise control. In part, the dexterity of the face and hand are due to the large amount of cortical space dedicated to their control. The precise sensory discrimination of the mouth and hand are due to the same disproportionate allocation of space. Inversion of the homunculus is clinically significant because the body parts represented on the medial aspect of the hemisphere receive their blood supply from one artery while those on the lateral surface receive theirs from another.

Transcortical Connections

The primary connection between the two hemispheres is provided by the corpus callosum, the largest fiber bundle in the nervous system. The corpus callosum forms the floor of the medial longitudinal fissure and the roof of the lateral ventricles. In crossing the midline, the corpus callosum connects functionally related areas in the two hemispheres.

Hemispheric Specialization

Historically, the cerebral hemispheres were viewed as mirror images of one another. The duplication of anatomy and physiology was justified on the basis of the crossed organization of the nervous system such that the right hemisphere controls the somatic and visceral functions of the left side of the body and the left hemisphere controls the right side. It was not until the corpus callosum (the major fiber bundle regulating communication between the two hemispheres) was sectioned that it became evident that the two hemispheres specialized in different functions (Fig. 19-3). In the absence of the corpus callosum, each hemisphere behaves as an individual brain with independent perception, learning, memory, thoughts, and emotional reactions, and neither is aware of the experiences of the other; literally, the right hand does not know what the left hand is doing.

The left hemisphere is characterized primarily by its specialization in language (speech, reading, writing) and is therefore operationally defined as the dominant hemisphere. Roughly 98 percent of the population has language controlled by the left hemisphere. The plenum temporal (the area of the temporal lobe specialized for speech) is larger in the left hemisphere by the 31st week of gestation, suggesting that this asymmetry does not develop in response to experience, but is innate. The left hemisphere also excels in intellectual, rational, verbal, and analytical thinking. It assumes primary control of analytical processes such as calculation, stereognosis (interpretation of sensory stimuli) from the right side of the body, audition from the right ear, vision from the right visual field, and olfaction from the left nostril.

The right hemisphere excels in perceiving and in emotional, nonverbal, and intuitive thinking. The right hemisphere also controls spatial orientation, nonverbal ideation, music appreciation, olfaction from the right nostril, audition from the left ear, vision from the left visual field, and stereognosis from the left side of the body. Because the right hemisphere usually does not control language, it is a more difficult hemisphere to evaluate. For example, in the absence of a corpus callosum, if a key is placed in an individual's left hand and vision is occluded, he or she can still interpret the sensory feedback and recognize the object. However, the object is recognized in the right hemisphere, and because the right hemisphere does not have the ability to produce speech, the individual cannot identify the object verbally. If asked to identify the test object by selecting from an array, the individual experiences no difficulty in selecting the key. The right hemisphere recognizes the object but does not have access to the left hemisphere, which would permit the individual to identify it verbally.

In a normally functioning brain, that is, a brain with an intact corpus callosum, each specialized region assumes primary responsibility for a particular aspect of the overall functional task. The results of specialized analyses are then shared freely among regions and hemispheres to enable individuals to perform a wide range of behaviors with no difficulty. In information processing parlance, this is called a parallel, distributed

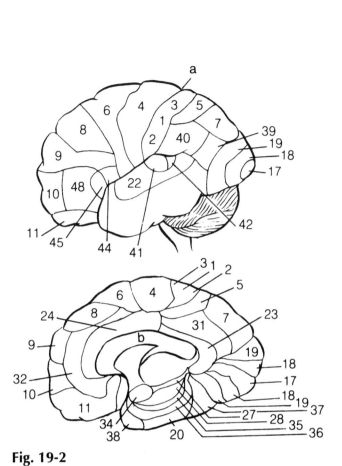

a
6
4
3
5
1
8
7
39
2
40
19
9
18
17
48
22
10
42
11
45
44
41
3
1
2
5
6
4
8
24
23
31
7
b
9
19
18
32
17
10
18
19
37
11
27
28
35
34
36
38
20

Fig. 19-2

Visual field
L
R
L-left
R-right
Olfaction
L
Olfaction
R
Speech writing
Stereognosis
R
b
Stereognosis
L
Audition
R L
Audition
L R
Main language
center
Spatial orientation
Calculation
Nonverbal ideation
Visual field
R
Visual field
L

Fig. 19-3

a	Central sulcus
	Cortical projection regions
	Primary motor (4)
	Secondary motor (6)
	Frontal eye field (8)
	Broca's area (44, 45)
	Primary somatosensory (3, 1, 2)
	Secondary somatosensory (5)
	Occipital eye field (19)
	Primary visual (17)
	Wernicke's area (22)
	Olfactory (38)
b	Corpus callosum

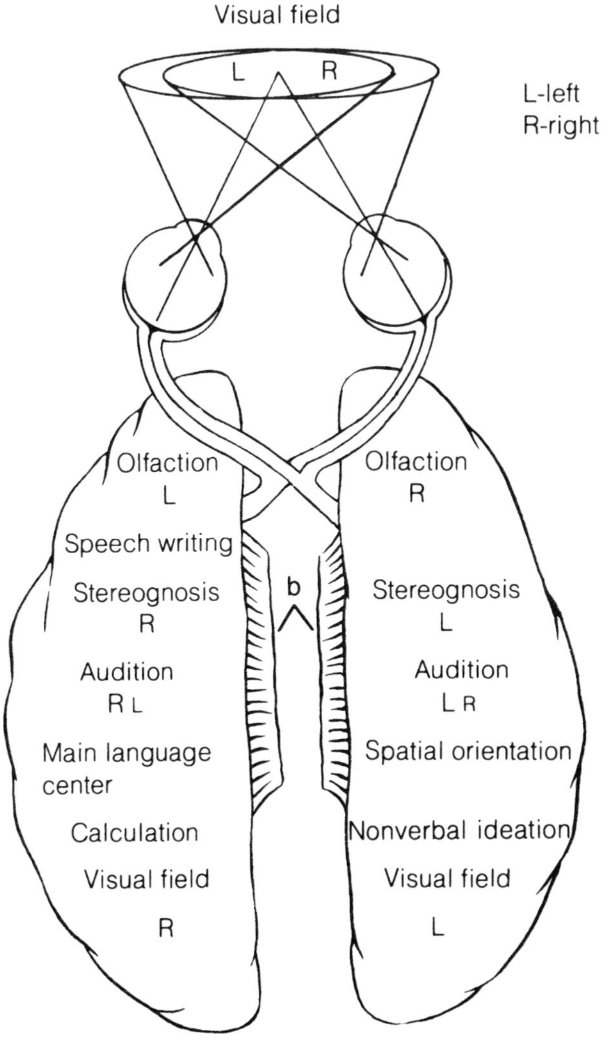

control system, that is, a task is broken down into components, with each component sent to a specialized center for analysis. Once complete, the results are freely shared among centers. Because each of the centers operates independently, they can all work on their part of the larger task, at the same time greatly speeding resolution time.

Clinical Aspects

Cerebrovascular accidents (CVA) also provide a means for studying the function of the cerebral cortex. Cerebrovascular accidents or strokes may occur in any vascular territory in the brain. The behavioral dysfunction that accompanies the stroke will depend on which areas of the brain are affected. Figure 19-4 shows the type of dysfunction suffered after damage to individual regions throughout the cerebral hemisphere.

Because the longitudinal systems connecting the brain and body are crossed, the symptoms and signs of CVA are seen on the side opposite the lesion. Because the right and left hemispheres specialize in controlling different functions, right and left CVAs produce very different clinical manifestations. Table 19-1 lists the behaviors attributed to the right and left hemispheres, and Table 19-2 lists deficits following right and left CVAs.

At birth the brain is already genetically predisposed to acquire language because of the presence of Wernicke's area (22) in the left hemisphere. This area is concerned with the comprehension of spoken and written language. If Wernicke's area is damaged, a receptive aphasia, commonly referred to as word deafness, is produced. In this type of aphasia, the auditory apparatus functions perfectly but the sounds being sensed are not perceived as language. This aphasia may also affect speech production because individuals are unable to understand their own spoken words. If the angular gyrus (area 39), which connects the visual cortex with Wernicke's area, is damaged, the individual experiences a visual word deafness (alexia) wherein the visual apparatus is functioning perfectly but written language is not perceived. This type of aphasia may be accompanied by an inability to write language (agraphia).

Speech production is also controlled in the left hemisphere in Broca's area (44 and 45). Damage in this area results in a productive aphasia characterized by impaired ability to produce verbal language. The motor apparatus for speech is intact, language is heard and perceived, and organized thought processes occur, but coherent verbal self-expression is impossible. Rhythmic speech, as in singing, seems to be a special case: It is specifically controlled in area 45; therefore, normal speech may be absent but singing is still possible. Mel Tillis is a male vocalist who stutters when speaking but does not stutter when singing.

The functions controlled by the cerebral cortex are dependent on the integrated output of columns of cells rather than the actions of any single neuron. This point is well illustrated by a clinical example. Convulsive activity is produced by changes in the collective properties of large numbers of cortical neurons. The electroencephalogram (EEG) uses electrodes applied to the scalp to record the activity of many cortical neurons simultaneously and is the best clinical tool for examining global cortical activity. Epileptic seizures are the direct result of abnormal, synchronized discharge of a large number of cortical neurons as seen on EEG. Synchronization of these normally independently discharging units produces stereotyped and involuntary changes in behavior, including transient loss of awareness, jerking movements, and possibly massive convulsions and loss of consciousness. Normally, lateral or surround inhibition of columns of cortical neurons prevents independently discharging units from becoming synchronized. Lateral or surround inhibition is created when a neuron or column of neurons facilitate

Table 19-1 Behaviors Controlled by Each Hemisphere

Behavior	Left Hemisphere	Right Hemisphere
Perception/cognition	Processing and producing language	Processing nonverbal stimuli (complex shapes, sounds, speech inflection)
		Visual-spatial perception
		Drawing inferences, integrating information
Information processing	Linear, sequential	Simultaneous, holistic
Cognitive style	Observing and analyzing details	Grasping overall organization or gestalt, sees patterns
Academic skills	Reading: word recognition, sound-symbol relationships, reading comprehension	Mathematical reasoning/judgment
	Performing mathematical calculations	Alignment of numbers in calculations
Motor	Movement sequencing	Sustaining a movement or posture
	Performing movements or gestures on command	
Emotions	Expression of positive emotions	Expression of negative emotions
		Perception of emotions

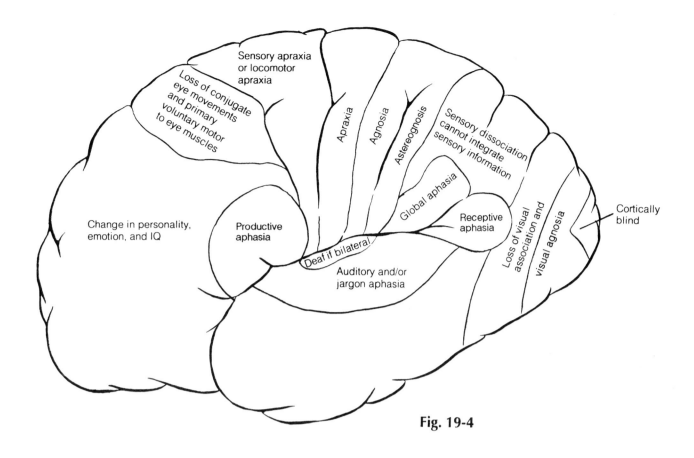

Fig. 19-4

Table 19-2   Deficits Following Cerebrovascular Accident

	Left Hemiplegia	Right Hemiplegia
Lesion	Right hemisphere	Left hemisphere
General deficits	Spatial, global	Language, temporal ordering
Visual-perceptual deficits	Left unilateral neglect (in some cases)	Motor apraxia
	Hand-eye coordination	Ideational apraxia
	Figure-ground discrimination	
	Spatial relations	
	Body image	
	Form constancy	
	Dressing apraxia	
	Constructional apraxia	
	Illusions of shortening of time	
Behavioral and intellectual deficits	Poor judgment, unrealistic expectations	Difficulty initiating tasks
	Denial of disability	Sequencing deficits
	Impulsive behavior	Processing delays
	Inability to abstract	Directional difficulties
	Rigidity of thought	Low frustration levels
	Impaired self-correction	Verbal and manual preservation
	Affect and emotional lability	Compulsive behavior
	Feelings of persecution	Extreme distractibility
	Irritability, confusion	
	Short attention span	
	Appearance of lethargy	

themselves and inhibit adjacent neurons. This arrangement helps to clarify the message being transmitted by the neuron or column and prevent interference of "crosstalk" from adjacent neurons. During an epileptic seizure, this surround inhibition breaks down and the discharge of columns of cortical neurons becomes synchronized at the seizure frequency, thereby losing control of their normal function and producing the seizure behavior. Thus, epileptic seizures are disorders of the cerebral cortex.

Abnormal discharge patterns of cortical neurons may be caused by many factors: trauma, oxygen deprivation, tumors, infection, and toxic states. However, only about half the individuals with epilepsy have clearly demonstrable causes.

Depending on the size of the area recruited, epileptic seizures can be either partial or general. Both forms produce distinctive, abnormal EEG patterns called spikes. Partial seizures begin from a focal center and spread to adjacent cortical regions by recruiting cells to beat at the seizure frequency. The area of the cortex involved in the abnormal discharge pattern will determine the associated behavioral activity. If the seizure involves the motor cortex, the individual will exhibit abnormal motor activity. Consciousness, visual, or auditory areas experiencing an abnormal discharge pattern will produce abnormal consciousness, visual, or auditory perceptions, respectively. Within a given cortical region, the body part with the largest representation is the most likely to be involved in the seizure activity. For example, the largest part of the motor homunculus is dedicated to the hand and face and they are also the most common body parts involved in motor seizures. The spread of partial seizures appears to be limited by powerful postsynaptic hyperpolarization in the cortex. During a generalized epileptic seizure, the abnormal discharge activity is evident over the entire brain at seizure onset and may result from an abnormal input originating in the brain stem reticular formation.

A common strategy for the medical management of seizure disorders is the administration of a generalized depressant such as phenytoin (Dilantin). The drug makes it more difficult for each neuron to reach discharge threshold, thereby making it more difficult to produce pathologically synchronized discharge of cortical cells.

20 Vascular System

Overview

Because the nervous system is incapable of storing essential nutrients (oxygen, glucose) yet has one of the highest metabolic rates of any organ in the body, continuous circulation of blood is essential for the sustained health and proper functioning of neural tissue. The vascular system provides the anatomy for the circulation of blood. If circulation is interrupted for even short periods of time, individual structures and the systems within which they operate begin to exhibit signs of alteration in function. Prolonged occlusion of circulation results in disease and death to the affected tissue. This infarction is referred to as a stroke or cerebrovascular accident and is accompanied by specific neurological signs and symptoms that correspond to the functions controlled by the damaged area.

Metabolism in the nervous system is aerobic or oxidative, and therefore requires a constant supply of oxygen. Although the brain constitutes only 2 percent of body weight, it receives 15 percent of cardiac output and uses 20 percent of the oxygen consumed by the body at rest. Metabolic needs, both the delivery of nutrients and removal of by-products, are met by the cerebrovascular system.

Anatomy of Cerebral Arteries

The cerebral arterial system consists of carotid and vertebrobasilar divisions, both of which emanate from the aortic arch (Fig. 20-1). The carotid system supplies arterial blood to the vast majority of the cerebral hemispheres. It is derived from the left and right internal carotid arteries, with each cerebral hemisphere being supplied by the ipsilateral internal carotid artery. Both internal carotid arteries enter the ventral surface of the brain immediately adjacent to the optic chiasm (Fig. 20-2A, B). After passing through the carotid canal located in the petrous portion of the temporal bone, each internal carotid artery bifurcates into anterior and middle cerebral arteries. The anterior cerebral artery branches profusely through the medial longitudinal fissure and supplies the inferior surface of the frontal lobe and medial aspect of the frontal and parietal lobes, as well as the anterior corpus callosum (Fig. 20-2C). Smaller penetrating branches supply the deeper cerebrum, diencephalon, limbic structures, head of the caudate nucleus, and anterior limb of the internal capsule (Fig. 20-3). The middle cerebral artery ascends through the lateral fissure and supplies blood to almost the entire lateral surface of the hemisphere, including motor, sensory, auditory, association, and speech areas of the frontal, parietal, occipital, and temporal lobes as well as the insula (see Fig. 20-2A, D). Important penetrating branches of the middle cerebral artery, the lenticulo-striate arteries, supply the putamen, outer globus pallidus, body of the caudate nucleus, and posterior limb of the internal capsule (Fig. 20-3).

The vertebrobasilar system supplies the brain stem and inferior surface of the temporal and occipital lobes (see Fig. 20-2A). Each vertebral artery arises from a subclavian artery, enters the cranium through the foramen magnum, and gives off two branches. The first descends and forms the anterior spinal artery while the second forms the posterior inferior cerebellar artery. The vertebral arteries ascend along the anterior surface of the medulla to the junction of the medulla and pons, where they join to form the basilar artery. The basilar artery ascends along the anterior surface of the pons, giving rise to the anterior inferior cerebellar arteries, inferior auditory arteries, and superior cerebellar arteries as it ascends. At the top of the pons, the basilar artery bifurcates, giving rise to the posterior cerebral arteries, which supply the inferior surface of the temporal lobes, inferior and medial surfaces of the occipital lobes, and posterior corpus callosum. Smaller penetrating branches of the posterior cerebral arteries supply parts of the thalamus, subthalamic nuclei, and midbrain (Fig. 20-3).

The choroidal arteries arise from both the carotid and vertebrobasilar systems. The anterior choroidal artery arises from the middle cerebral artery and supplies the choroid plexus of the lateral ventricles, hippocampus, and parts of the globus pallidus and posterior limb of the internal capsule. The posterior choroidal artery arises from the posterior cerebral artery and supplies the choroid plexus of the third ventricle and dorsal surface of the thalamus.

Throughout the cerebral arterial system, pressure is equalized by a series of anastomoses (communication between two vessels). The circle of Willis is probably the largest and best-known anastomosis in the brain (see Fig. 20-2B). It plays an important part in equalizing the pressure and distributing the blood from the carotid and vertebrobasilar systems. The anterior communicating artery connects the left and right anterior cerebral arteries, and the posterior communicating artery connects the middle and posterior cerebral arteries in each hemisphere.

Clinical Aspects

Reversible (ischemic) and irreversible (infarction) changes in cell function can be traced directly to the availability of oxygen. Oxygen depletion results in an almost immediate alteration in cellular metabolism (a decrease in oxygen corresponds to a decrease in discharge frequency). Under ischemic conditions, metabolism is accelerated and glucose is quickly depleted.

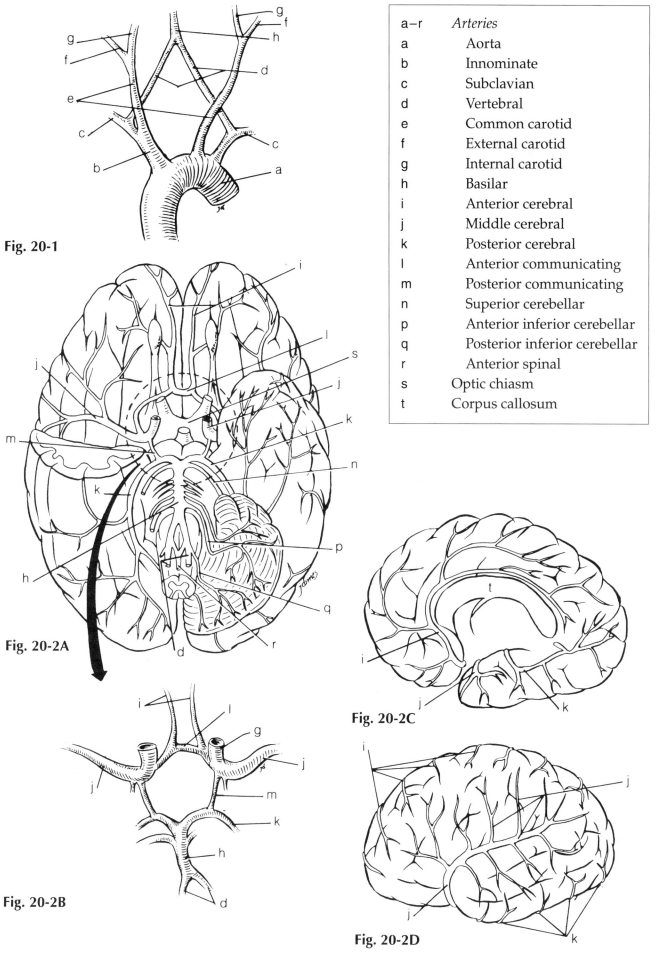

Fig. 20-1

a–r	Arteries
a	Aorta
b	Innominate
c	Subclavian
d	Vertebral
e	Common carotid
f	External carotid
g	Internal carotid
h	Basilar
i	Anterior cerebral
j	Middle cerebral
k	Posterior cerebral
l	Anterior communicating
m	Posterior communicating
n	Superior cerebellar
p	Anterior inferior cerebellar
q	Posterior inferior cerebellar
r	Anterior spinal
s	Optic chiasm
t	Corpus callosum

Fig. 20-2A

Fig. 20-2B

Fig. 20-2C

Fig. 20-2D

141

Potassium is lost rapidly from inside the cell, as the concentration of extracellular potassium increases and membrane potential and the ability to generate and conduct nerve impulses are lost.

Reversible ischemic episodes (transient ischemic attacks) are attributed to a temporary vasospasm or occlusion in a cerebral vessel. Symptoms have a rapid onset, last for a matter of minutes or hours, and are completely reversible, with no aftereffects or residual deficits. Transient ischemic attacks are a reliable predictor of impending stroke within the following six months to a year.

In the normal brain, cerebral blood flow is regulated automatically in response to changes in arterial blood pressure and local metabolic demands. The brain accomplishes this autoregulation through myogenic, neurogenic, and chemometabolic mechanisms. Smooth muscle in the walls of cerebral blood vessels is capable of causing a vasoconstriction or dilation and thereby an increase or decrease in blood pressure, respectively. Neurogenic mechanisms include autonomic regulation of myogenic function through chemoreceptors within the brain. Stimulation of sympathetic fibers produces vasoconstriction and a decrease in cerebral blood flow. Stimulation of parasympathetic fibers produces vasodilation and an increase in cerebral blood flow. Chemometabolic factors exert a strong influence on cerebral blood flow. Carbon dioxide is the most potent physiological and pharmacological agent to influence cerebral blood flow. Any increase in the local carbon dioxide concentration (PCO_2) causes rapid vasodilation and increase in cerebral blood flow, while a decrease in carbon dioxide concentration produces vasoconstriction and a decrease in cerebral blood flow. Alterations in the brain hydrogen ion concentration (pH) are also powerful chemometabolic factors. A decrease in brain pH (acidosis) due to any cause will produce vasodilation and an increase in cerebral blood flow, whereas an increase in brain pH (alkalosis) will produce vasoconstriction and a reduction in cerebral blood flow. Abundance of lactic acid produced by a shift to anabolic metabolism in the region of ischemia is a potent vasodilator.

When an occlusion occurs in a cerebral vessel, a regional ischemia develops because of the reduction in available blood supply. Responses to the ischemia include a decrease in blood pressure beyond the occlusion, interruption of the oxygen supply, increase in the carbon dioxide concentration, and lactic acidosis. Together these factors produce vasodilation and increased cerebral blood flow in the ischemic region. These responses will increase regional blood flow and may prevent infarction or reduce the area of greatest damage. Within seconds the ischemic cell begins to swell. If its metabolic needs are not met soon, irreversible damage occurs within minutes. The resultant death and destruction of cells increase the water content in the surrounding tissue. The associated brain edema (fluid swelling) further impairs the function of cells in the region surrounding the infarct. When the condition has reached equilibrium (through whatever means) and the cellular debris is removed, a cavity remains.

The most common causes of deprivation of adequate blood supply to the brain (cerebrovascular accident) are thrombosis and embolism. Both thrombosis (development of a blood clot or thrombus) and embolism (obstruction of a blood vessel by a foreign body, clot, air, fat, or tumor) interrupt blood supply by occlusion that produces ischemia and hematoma (tumor or swelling containing blood). The ischemia and resulting damage following occlusion are dependent on available collateral flow. The most damaging results of vascular occlusion are produced by the mechanical effects of the hematoma.

Middle Cerebral Artery Syndrome

The middle cerebral artery is the most common site of cerebrovascular accident. If the stroke occurs close to the vessel's origin, the symptoms are severe and very disabling. Middle cerebral artery syndrome includes a contralateral weakness (hemiplegia), hemisensory deficit, homonymous hemianopia, and, depending on the hemisphere involved, either aphasia if the dominant hemisphere is involved or impaired spatial perception if the nondominant hemisphere is involved. Muscle tone is usually decreased at first (hypotonia or flaccidity) but gradually increases over days or weeks to spasticity with increased deep tendon reflexes. Sensory deficits are most severe for proprioceptive and discriminative modalities. Impairments include two-point discrimination, the ability to recognize objects by their sensory qualities (stereognosis), and perception of a touch stimulus if another is presented simultaneously to the uninvolved extremity (extinction). The arm and particularly the hand are usually involved more than the leg, but not in every case. When the deep penetrating vessels supplying the internal capsule are involved, the face, hand, and foot are afflicted equally. Destruction of lateral corticospinal tract fibers accounts for the prominent involvement of the hand, while the loss of corticobulbar fibers projecting to cranial nerves accounts for facial involvement. The involvement of upper motor neurons is reflected in a positive Babinski sign, which is usually present from the onset.

Depending on the hemisphere involved, the syndrome includes either disturbance of language or impaired spatial perception. Lesion of the left opercular (perisylvian) cortex produces aphasia. Lesion of the frontal opercular region (Broca's area, 45 of Brodmann) produces difficulty with speech production and writing while preserving speech comprehension (productive aphasia). Lesion of the posterior superior temporal gyrus (Wernicke's area, 22) produces difficulty with speech comprehension and reading (receptive aphasia). Extensive opercular damage may produce a particularly disabling global aphasia (a combination of productive and receptive aphasia).

Lesion of the right middle cerebral artery produces difficulties with spatial perception, including copying

a	Territory of the anterior cerebral artery
b	Territory of the middle cerebral artery
c	Territory of the posterior cerebral artery
d	Territory of the penetrating branches of the middle cerebral artery (lateral striate artery)
e	Territory of the anterior choroidal artery (medial striate artery)

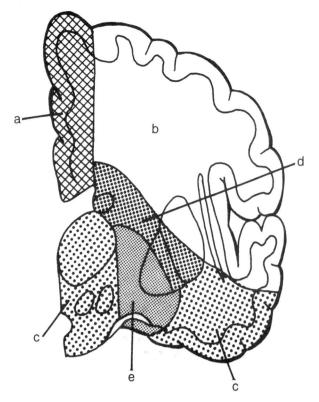

Fig. 20-3

simple diagrams (constructional apraxia) and dressing (dressing apraxia). Apraxia is difficulty in performing learned movements in the absence of loss of power, sensation, or coordination. Clients may fail to recognize their hemiplegia (anosognosia), the left side of their body (hemineglect), or any external object left of their own midline (hemi-inattention).

Anterior Cerebral Artery Syndrome

Lesion of the anterior cerebral artery causes hemiparesis and sensory deficits in the contralateral lower extremity. Effects are similar to those found following lesion of the middle cerebral artery but restricted to the lower extremity due to the somatotopic organization of the cerebral cortex. Bilateral lesion of the anterior cerebral artery may also produce profound changes in personality, including apathy, akinesia, and muteness.

Posterior Cerebral Artery Syndrome

The symptoms associated with lesion of the posterior cerebral artery are contralateral homonymous hemianopia with or without a hemiparesis. Thalamic involvement may produce contralateral hemisensory disturbances including spontaneous pain and dysesthesia (thalamic pain syndrome). Involvement of the subthalamic nucleus may cause severe chorea in the proximal segments of the contralateral upper extremity (hemiballism). Bilateral lesion may cause cortical blindness and memory disorders. However, posterior cerebral artery syndrome is quite variable because of several anastomotic connections with the middle cerebral artery that vary between individuals.

Lacunar Syndrome

The smaller penetrating arteries that originate from the larger vessels are particularly susceptible to damage caused by hypertension. Because these vessels lack anastomotic interconnections, occlusion of individual vessels causes small (less than 1.5 cm in diameter) strokes (lacunes). A lacune in the internal capsule that affects only corticospinal fibers will cause pure contralateral hemiparesis with little or no sensory loss. A lacune in the ventral posterior nucleus of the thalamus produces a pure contralateral sensory loss with little or no motor, visual, language, or spatial disturbance. Most lacunes are asymptomatic; however, if bilateral and numerous, they may cause a characteristic syndrome (état lacunaire), which includes progressive dementia, shuffling gait, and pseudobulbar palsy.

Brain Stem Syndromes

Most brain stem strokes follow occlusion of the vertebral or basilar arteries and the resulting symptoms and signs are variable; however, two classic syndromes exist. Lateral medullary (Wallenberg) syndrome results from lesion of large branches of the vertebral or basilar arteries supplying the lateral brain stem and cerebellum. Symptoms usually include loss of pain and temperature sensation on the ipsilateral face and contralateral body, ipsilateral limb ataxia, vertigo, nystagmus, and Horner's syndrome with ipsilateral ptosis, miosis, dilation of facial blood vessels, and facial anhidrosis (lack of sweating). Medial brain stem syndrome results from lesion of the penetrating branches of the basilar or vertebral arteries in the caudal pons. Symptoms usually include ipsilateral abducens palsy (medial deviation of the eye) and a contralateral hemiplegia.

Hemorrhagic Lesions

Hemorrhage accounts for approximately 20 percent of cerebrovascular accidents, while occlusion (thrombolic and embolic) accounts for 70 percent. Hemorrhage may occur in any of the cerebral arteries and is associated with hypertension. Cerebral hemorrhage has a rapid onset and destroys brain tissue through anoxia and the occlusive pressure produced by the hematoma. Because of the nature of the lesion and the resulting damage, unless hemorrhagic lesions receive prompt medical attention, they are frequently fatal. Even in the presence of medical attention, they are associated with a high mortality. Bleeding within the meninges (subdural hemorrhage) causes brain tissue to shift off the midline to the side opposite the hemorrhage because of increased pressure. The shifting brain tissue may herniate through the tentorium into the midbrain (transtentorial or uncal hernia) and produce a decorticate lesion (separate the cortex from the brain stem). If the hemorrhage is massive and the pressure great enough, brain stem tissue may herniate through the foramen magnum into the spinal canal and produce a decerebrate lesion (separate the brain stem from the spinal cord). Both are potentially life-threatening conditions.

Cerebrovascular accidents, or strokes, may occur in any vascular territory in the brain. The behavioral dysfunction that accompanies the stroke will depend on which areas in the brain are affected. Figure 19-4 illustrates the type of symptoms frequently suffered after damage to individual regions throughout the cerebral hemisphere.

Venous Drainage of the Brain

Veins of the brain have thin walls that contain no smooth muscle or valves. They cross the subarachnoid space to join the dural venous sinus system. The venous drainage of the brain is divided into superficial and deep systems (Fig. 20-4). The superficial system is located in the subarachnoid space and follows the contour of the hemispheres, with major vessels protected inside the medial longitudinal and lateral fissures. The superior sagittal sinus follows the medial longitudinal fissure and drains blood from the cortex and superior white matter located near the midline. It empties directly into the transverse sinuses. The

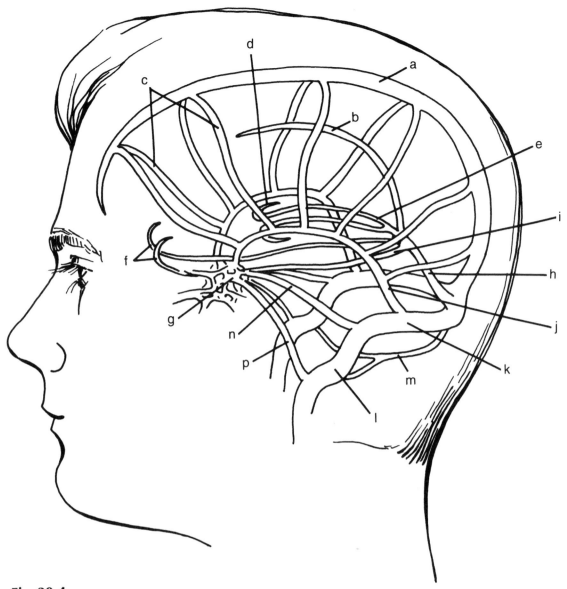

Fig. 20-4

a	Superior sagittal sinus
b	Inferior sagittal sinus
c	Superior anastomotic veins
d	Thalamostriate vein
e	Internal cerebral vein
f	Anterior cerebral vein
g	Cavernous sinus
h	Straight sinus
i	Basal vein
j	Inferior anastomotic vein
k	Transverse sinus
l	Sigmoid sinus
m	Occipital sinuses
n	Superior petrosal sinus
p	Inferior petrosal sinus

superficial middle cerebral vein follows the lateral fissure and drains blood from the superficial region of the lateral aspect of the hemisphere. It empties into the transverse sinus via the inferior anastomotic vein. The superior sagittal sinus and superficial middle cerebral veins are connected by anastomotic veins running between the two.

The deep venous system drains blood from the deep white matter and nuclei of the brain. The internal cerebral vein drains the deep parts of its hemisphere originating as the thalamostriate and choroid veins. Numerous smaller veins join to form the internal cerebral vein as it courses below the corpus callosum and empties into the straight sinus via the great cerebral vein. The basal vein drains the inferior and medial aspects of its hemisphere. It originates as the anterior cerebral vein, which accompanies the anterior cerebral artery. It is then joined by the deep middle cerebral vein and several smaller veins as it courses posteriorly and empties into the straight sinus via the great ventral vein. The inferior sagittal sinus drains the medial aspect of the cerebral hemispheres superior to the internal cerebral vein and empties into the transverse sinuses by way of the straight sinus. The transverse sinuses are continuous with the sigmoid sinuses, which return the blood to general circulation by way of the jugular veins. The cavernous sinus drains blood from the region of the hypothalamus and empties into the sigmoid sinuses and jugular veins via the superior and inferior petrosal sinuses.

Clinical Aspects

There are no common clinical problems associated with venous drainage of the brain.

Arterial Supply to the Spinal Cord

In the spinal cord, arterial blood is supplied by one anterior and two posterior arteries, which extend the length of the spinal cord (Fig. 20-5). The anterior spinal artery is located in the anterior medial fissure. It arises from a small descending branch of each vertebral artery that unites and descends along the ventral surface of the pons, medulla, and cervical spinal cord. In the thoracic, lumbar, and sacral regions, blood is supplied by a series of radicular arteries (root-like beginning of arteries) that arise outside the central nervous system. The junction between spinal and radicular arteries creates two zones (upper thoracic and lumbar levels) where the spinal cord is most susceptible to ischemia (local and temporary reduction in blood flow due to obstruction of circulation). Caudally, the anterior spinal artery also serves the cauda equina. At each segmental level, sulcal branches from the anterior spinal artery penetrate and supply the anterior two thirds of the spinal cord, including the lateral horns, anterior horns, and anterior funiculi, bilaterally.

The posterior spinal arteries are paired structures. Each arises from a small branch of the ipsilateral vertebral artery and extends the length of the spinal cord adjacent to the posterior lateral sulcus. A series of posterior radicular arteries contribute to posterior spinal arteries in the thoracic, lumbar, and sacral regions. The posterior spinal arteries distribute blood to the posterior one third of the spinal cord, including the posterior horns and posterior funiculi, bilaterally.

Clinical Aspects

Vascular disease of the spinal cord is usually restricted to the anterior spinal artery where, because of its distribution, it impairs motor function as well as sensation of pain and temperature below the level of the lesion while leaving the other sensory modalities unaffected.

Venous Drainage of the Spinal Cord

The venous drainage of the spinal cord has a distribution similar to that of the arterial supply (Fig. 20-5). Like the arterial system, a variable number of anterior and posterior radicular veins form the basis of the system. The anterior radicular veins form a distinct anterior medial vein and paired anterolateral trunks that extend the length of the spinal cord. The posterior radicular veins form a posterior medial vein as well as smaller, paired posterolateral trunks that extend the length of the spinal cord. As with the arteries, a meningeal plexus of veins connects the longitudinal trunks. From the anterior spinal vein, sulcal branches pass through the anterior medial fissure, where they drain blood from the lateral horns, anterior horns, and anterior funiculi, bilaterally. Sulcal branches from the posterior radicular veins also drain the posterior horns and posterior funiculi, bilaterally.

Clinical Aspects

There are no common clinical problems associated with venous drainage of the spinal cord.

Vascular Supply and Clinical Aspects of Peripheral Nerves

The arterial blood supply to peripheral nerves is derived from rich anastomotic plexuses of small penetrating arterioles that originate from peripheral arteries of the body (Fig. 20-5). Small branches from peripheral arteries penetrate the protective covering of the nerve and project longitudinally inside of the nerve. Different regional arteries form anastomotic chains within the peripheral nerve that extend the length of the nerve. Because of the rich anastomosis derived from several different sources, ischemic vascular disease of peripheral nerves is rare. When it occurs, such disease is usually due to direct compression of a nerve.

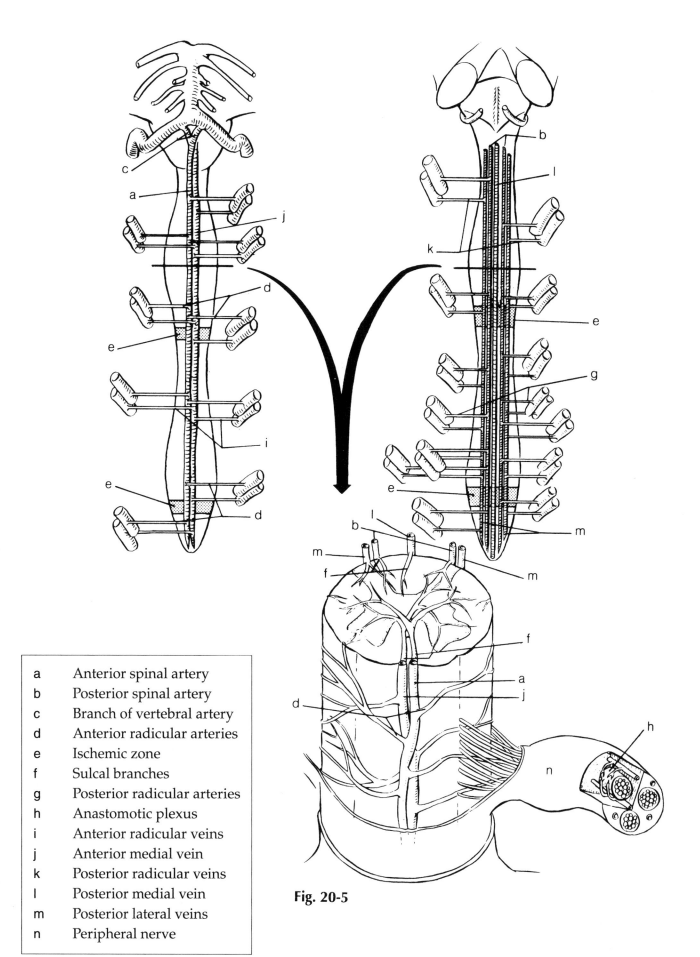

a	Anterior spinal artery
b	Posterior spinal artery
c	Branch of vertebral artery
d	Anterior radicular arteries
e	Ischemic zone
f	Sulcal branches
g	Posterior radicular arteries
h	Anastomotic plexus
i	Anterior radicular veins
j	Anterior medial vein
k	Posterior radicular veins
l	Posterior medial vein
m	Posterior lateral veins
n	Peripheral nerve

Fig. 20-5

21 Ventricular and Cerebrospinal Fluid Systems

Overview

The ventricles are part of a system of caverns that extend throughout the central nervous system. Cerebrospinal fluid is produced in and circulates through these caverns, supporting metabolism and acting as a hydraulic buffer to protect nervous tissue.

Structure

The central nervous system developed from a hollow neural tube. In the mature brain, remnants of the neural tube remain as a cavernous system that changed its shape along with the developing nervous system. Components of this system of caverns (the ventricular system) exist in each region of the brain and spinal cord, and retain direct contact with one another (Fig. 21-1). The forebrain contains the lateral ventricles (one in each hemisphere) and the third ventricle. The lateral ventricles are continuous with the third ventricle by way of the interventricular foramina of Monro. The cerebral aqueduct traverses the midbrain and leads from the third to the fourth ventricle, which is located in the hindbrain between the brain stem and cerebellum. The fourth ventricle is continuous with the central canal of the spinal cord.

The lateral ventricles are much larger than the third and fourth ventricles. They follow the contour of the forebrain such that they extend to all four lobes: anterior horns in the frontal lobe, bodies in the parietal lobe, posterior horns in the occipital lobe, and inferior horns in the temporal lobe. The third ventricle is located directly in the midline, with right and left thalami forming the lateral walls. The fourth ventricle is diamond-shaped with an inferior projection that is continuous, for a short distance, with the central canal of the spinal cord. In the mature spinal cord, the central canal is discontinuous if not completely closed.

The ventricular system opens into the subarachnoid space via three foramina of the fourth ventricle. Two smaller foramina of Luschka are located laterally and one larger foramen of Magendie is located on the midline of the posterior wall (Fig. 21-2). The subarachnoid space also envelops spinal and cranial nerves such that these nerves are bathed in cerebrospinal fluid as they exit the central nervous system.

Cerebrospinal fluid is a clear substance produced by the choroid plexus and found in each ventricle. The choroid plexus consists of a rich bed of capillaries that mix with the pia mater lining the walls of the ventricular system and is the primary producer of cerebrospinal fluid. There are two large plexuses, one located on the floor of each lateral ventricle, and smaller ones found on the roofs of the third and fourth ventricles. The nervous system contains approximately 125 ml cerebrospinal fluid, which is completely replaced several times a day.

Cerebrospinal fluid circulates constantly throughout the ventricles and subarachnoid space at a slow pace. The general direction of flow is from the lateral ventricles through the intervertebral foramina to the third ventricle, on through the cerebral aqueduct to the fourth ventricle, and out through the foramina of Luschka and Magendie into the subarachnoid space (Fig. 21-2). Once into the subarachnoid space, there are two general patterns of flow. The route of greater importance proceeds rostrally around the cerebellum and cerebral hemispheres and into the medial longitudinal fissure. Ultimately cerebrospinal fluid exits through valve-like tubules in the arachnoid villi (arachnoid granulation) into the great venous sinuses of the dura mater and becomes absorbed by the venous system, especially the superior sagittal sinus. The route of lesser importance proceeds caudally through the foramen magnum and subarachnoid space surrounding the spinal cord, where it is partially reabsorbed by the leptomeninges.

Function

Cerebrospinal fluid has several functions. First, it helps maintain homeostasis in the central nervous system. Because the constituents of cerebrospinal fluid are in equilibrium with brain extracellular fluid, it helps to maintain a stable external environment for the central nervous system. Second, while circulating in the subarachnoid space, cerebrospinal fluid provides buoyancy to the central nervous system, decreasing the weight of the brain on the skull. Third, it acts as a hydraulic shock absorber, protecting delicate neural tissue from impact with its bony covering. Fourth, it acts as a fluid transport system by which chemical substances circulate throughout the central nervous system to deliver nutrients and remove metabolites. This is important because the central nervous system has few if any lymphatic vessels.

Clinical Aspects

For diagnostic purposes, cerebrospinal fluid is drawn either from a lumbar (L4–L5 most commonly) or cervical (C1–C2 less commonly) puncture using a hypodermic syringe (spinal tap). Examination of cerebrospinal fluid includes checks for cellular composition and pressure. The presence of more than six white cells per cubic millimeter or any red cells is of pathological significance. Normal pressure is as follows: newborns, 30 to 80 mm H_2O; children, 50 to 100 mm; adults, 75 to 150 mm. Increased pressure may be observed in patients with numerous pathologies involving hemorrhage or

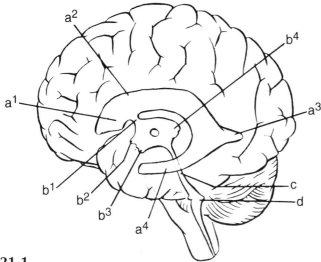

Fig. 21-1

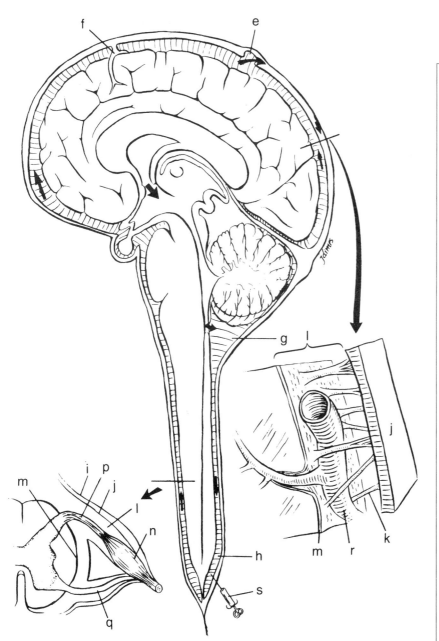

Fig. 21-2

a	Lateral ventricle
a^1	Anterior horn
a^2	Body
a^3	Posterior horn
a^4	Inferior horn
b	Third ventricle
b^1	Foramen of Monro
b^2	Preoptic recess
b^3	Infundibular recess
b^4	Pineal recess
c	Cerebral aqueduct
d	Fourth ventricle
d^1	Foramina of Luschka
d^2	Foramen of Magendie
e	Arachnoid granulation
f	Great venous sinus
g	Cisterna magna
h	Lumbar cistern
i	Dura mater
j	Arachnoid mater
k	Arachnoid trabecula
l	Subarachnoid space
m	Pia mater
n	Dorsal root ganglion
p	Dorsal root
q	Ventral root
r	Cerebral vessel
s	Hypodermic syringe

occlusion of cerebrospinal fluid systems, infection, head injury, metabolic encephalopathies, hydrocephalus, and intracranial hypertension. Decreased pressure may be caused by dehydration or occlusion of cerebrospinal fluid in the spinal canal.

Any obstruction to the normal passage of cerebrospinal fluid causes the fluid to back up in the ventricles and leads to a general increase in intracranial pressure. Because neural tissue is pliable, increases in intracranial pressure will produce noticeable changes in the location of some neural structures. Any shifts in neural tissue may be seen on sonography, computed tomography (CT), or magnetic resonance imaging (MRI). Increased intracranial pressure causes neural tissue to shift off the midline, moving in the direction opposite the increased pressure. The effects of increased intracranial pressure can also be seen by inspecting the fundus of the eye with an ophthalmoscope. Increased intracranial pressure produces a swelling of retinal veins and head of the optic nerve (papilledema). The most common cause of papilledema is a brain tumor.

Hydrocephalus is an increase in the volume of cerebrospinal fluid, usually within the ventricular system. Three types of hydrocephalus are common. Obstructive hydrocephalus is produced by an obstruction of the normal flow of cerebrospinal fluid out of the ventricles. Common sites of obstruction include the foramen of Monro, the cerebral aqueduct, and the foramina of Luschka or Magendie. Many types of pathology may cause obstructive hydrocephalus, including developmental abnormalities, brain tumors, and inflammatory processes. Communicating hydrocephalus is produced by free communication between the ventricles and subarachnoid space. Common causes include reabsorption of cerebrospinal fluid at the arachnoid villi and disturbance in the circulation through the subarachnoid space. The third type is compensatory hydrocephalus, noted as increased cerebrospinal fluid around a small brain (microcephaly) where the extra space between the cortex and skull is occupied by excess cerebrospinal fluid. In young children for whom the cranial sutures are unfused, hydrocephalus usually causes cranial enlargement. In older children and adults with hydrocephalus, the fused sutures will not permit cranial enlargement; therefore, the head is normal in size but intracranial pressure is elevated. Sustained increases in intracranial pressure often cause an increase in the size of the ventricles at the expense of the surrounding neural tissue. Children with hydrocephalus often fail to achieve mental and motor milestones while adults may experience lethargy, headaches, vomiting, and unsteady gait.

22 Consciousness System

Overview

The function of the consciousness system is to regulate the behavioral states of consciousness, attention, and sleep through specific changes in neuronal activity in the brain stem and basal forebrain that result in functional changes in thalamic and cortical circuits. The consciousness system is a diffuse multineuronal, polysynaptic system located in the brain stem, diencephalon, and cerebral hemispheres. Disorders of consciousness range from temporary conditions with no permanent aftereffects, such as fainting, to massive structural damage in both hemispheres of the brain stem that leads to brain death.

Anatomy

Structures of the consciousness system include portions of the brain stem reticular formation, the basal forebrain, neurochemically defined systems of the brain stem and forebrain, the thalamus, ascending projection pathways, and widespread areas of the cerebral cortex (Fig. 22-1).

The Reticular Formation

The reticular formation consists of multiple networks of nuclei and projection fibers that receive and integrate information from many areas of the neuraxis, including the somatic and visceral sensory systems, cerebral cortex, basal forebrain, hypothalamus, and cerebellum. It extends from the caudal medulla to the thalamus and basal forebrain area. The predominant organizational schema of the reticular formation is divergence, so that a single reticular neuron makes connections with many afferent neurons that project throughout the system. During development, the phylogenetically older reticular formation was surrounded by newer sensory and motor pathways serving specific functions (sometimes referred to as inner and outer tubes, respectively). Functionally, the reticular formation can be subdivided into medial and lateral portions. The medial portion is the output zone from which all efferent projections arise. The lateral portion is the input zone that receives afferents to the reticular formation.

The efferent pathways from the reticular formation contribute to the motor control and visceral control systems as well as reaching widespread areas of the cerebral cortex directly via the medial forebrain bundle and indirectly through thalamocortical projections (Fig. 22-2). Medial and lateral reticulospinal tracts exert influence directly onto lower motor neuron pools.

The reticular formation receives input from collateral branches of second-order neurons in the major somatic sensory systems (spinothalamic and lemniscal) as they pass through the brain stem; direct projections

from widespread areas of the cerebral cortex as well as collateral branches from corticobulbar and corticospinal tracts; fibers from other structures, including the cerebellum, basal ganglia, hypothalamus, cranial nerve nuclei, and superior and inferior colliculi; and visceral afferents from the spinal cord and cranial nerves (Fig. 22-3).

Neurochemically Defined Systems of the Brain Stem and Basal Forebrain

The consciousness system includes two subsystems defined by the chemistry of their neurotransmitter substance: cholinergic and monoaminergic systems (Table 22-1).

The cholinergic system includes direct cortical projections (neurons from the dorsal tegmentum, and basalis and septal nuclei of the basal forebrain via the medial forebrain bundle) and indirect cortical projections (neurons from the basal forebrain and mesopontine tegmentum via the medial thalamus and thalamocortical projections). Cholinergic input to the thalamic reticular nucleus modulates the activity of the thalamus and thalamocortical projections, making them more receptive to sensory input.

The monoaminergic system includes norepinephrine, serotonin, and histamine cell groups. The norepinephrine cells are located in the locus ceruleus. These cells increase their activity in response to new and challenging stimuli and thus are an important mechanism of arousal and attention and also paradoxical (rapid eye movement) sleep. The serotonin cells are located in the raphe nuclei. The rostral group of raphe nuclei (upper pons and midbrain) give rise to ascending fibers that project to the thalamus, hypothalamus, basal forebrain, and cerebral hemispheres. The caudal raphe nuclei (lower pons and medulla) give rise to descending fibers that project to other areas of the brain stem and spinal cord. The serotonergic system exerts influence on a widespread area of the central nervous system and facilitates sleep. The histamine neurons

Table 22-1. Neurochemically Defined Systems

Neurotransmitter	Location	Modulates
Acetylcholine	Dorsal tegmentum of pons and midbrain	Wakefulness
	Basal forebrain	Rapid eye movement (REM) sleep
Monoamines		
Norepinephrine	Locus ceruleus	Wakefulness, attention
Serotonin	Raphe nuclei	Non-REM sleep
Histamine	Hypothalamus	Wakefulness

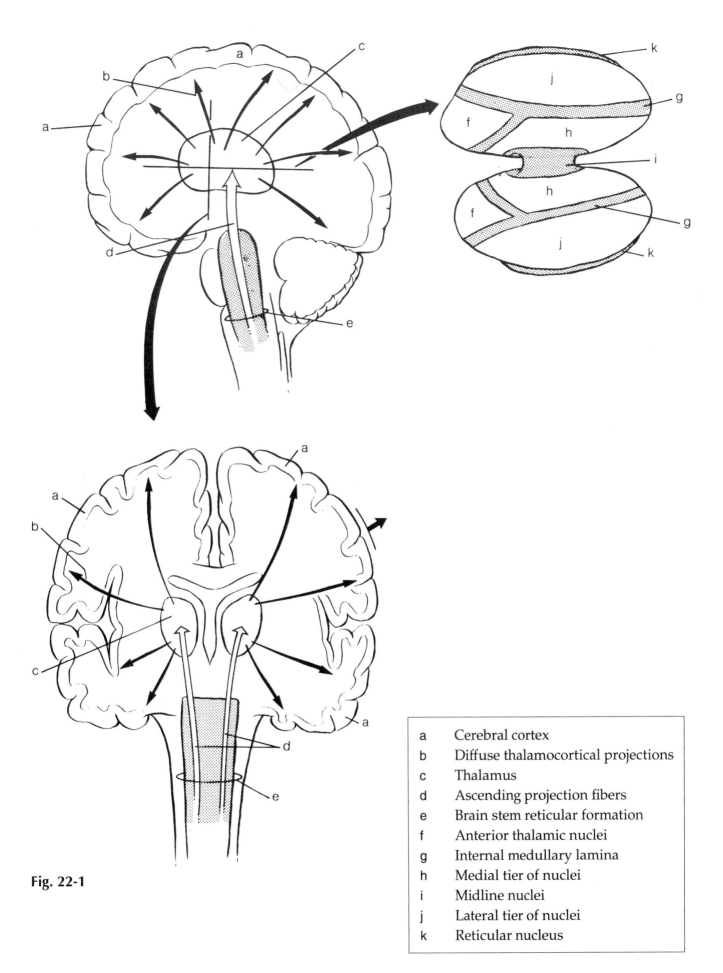

Fig. 22-1

a	Cerebral cortex
b	Diffuse thalamocortical projections
c	Thalamus
d	Ascending projection fibers
e	Brain stem reticular formation
f	Anterior thalamic nuclei
g	Internal medullary lamina
h	Medial tier of nuclei
i	Midline nuclei
j	Lateral tier of nuclei
k	Reticular nucleus

153

are located in the posterior lateral hypothalamus and enhance arousal and wakefulness.

Thalamus

The thalamus is an egg-shaped constellation of nuclei that acts as the final processing station where ascending information is organized before being transmitted to the cerebral cortex. The cortex also projects back to the thalamus so as to modulate what information it receives from the thalamus. Each thalamic nucleus contains interneurons and projection neurons. Functionally, the thalamus can be subdivided into specific and nonspecific nuclei. Specific nuclei are located lateral to the internal medullary lamina (a Y-shaped, myelinated fiber bundle subdividing the thalamus into anterior, medial, and lateral parts) and nonspecific nuclei are located medially. Specific thalamic nuclei receive somatotopically organized input from sensory and motor systems and have somatotopically organized reciprocal connections with specialized areas in the cerebral cortex. Nonspecific nuclei receive input from other thalamic nuclei, the reticular formation, and the basal forebrain and project to all areas of the cerebral cortex via the diffuse thalamic projection system. The nonspecific thalamic nuclei include the midline nuclei, intralaminar nuclei, and reticular nucleus. The reticular nucleus does not project to the cerebral cortex directly but is critical in regulating the activity of thalamocortical circuits. By regulating thalamocortical circuits the reticular system plays a critical role in regulating the activity of the cerebral cortex, thereby modifying levels of consciousness and alertness.

Basal Forebrain Area

The basal forebrain area is located on the ventral and medial aspect of the cerebral hemisphere and includes the nucleus basalis (basal nucleus of Meynert), septal nucleus, and rostral portion of the medial forebrain bundle (Fig. 22-4). The nucleus basalis is the major source of extrathalamic input to the cerebral cortex. Its neurons disperse cholinergic neurotransmitter substance to widespread areas of the cerebral cortex. The medial forebrain bundle is a major tract that runs from the midbrain tegmentum through the lateral hypothalamus into the septum, preoptic area, hypothalamus, basal olfactory region, and cingulate gyrus. This bundle is the most rostral projection of the reticular activating system and contains ascending and descending fibers that interconnect the brain stem and cortex. Many of the cholinergic and monoaminergic fibers that originate in the brain stem project to the cortex via this pathway.

Ascending Pathways to the Cerebral Cortex

Cortical input arising from specific thalamic nuclei is phasic because it originates as discrete sensory events (stimuli) in the internal or external environment. Cortical input arising from nonspecific thalamic nuclei and extrathalamic input originating from cholinergic and monoaminergic systems exert a tonic influence on cortical activity. Cholinergic and monoaminergic systems have widespread projections and are capable of producing global changes in cortical activity and behavior. All areas of the cerebral cortex appear to participate in consciousness and are considered to be part of the consciousness system.

Functions Controlled by the Consciousness System

The consciousness system is responsible for controlling consciousness, attention, and the wake-sleep states.

Consciousness

Consciousness is a subjective state that involves an awareness of self and the environment. It implies a state of arousal and alertness in which changing stimuli from the internal and external environments are perceived and responded to adaptively. There are two aspects of arousal and consciousness: the overall level of activity in the cerebral cortex and the activity in the reticular activating system and its projections. The reticular system receives sensory input via collateral branches from every major sensory pathway, which keeps the reticular activating system in a constant state of activation that in turn activates the cortex to maintain wakefulness. The tonic state of activation maintained in the reticular activating system and cerebral cortex is dependent upon neurons in the locus ceruleus, basal forebrain, mesopontine tegmentum, and lateral hypothalamus.

Attention

The degree of overall attention to the environment and perception of specific sensory events is also determined by the consciousness system. The cholinergic neurons of the basal forebrain facilitate the ability of the cerebral cortex to process sensory information. The basal forebrain can cause localized or generalized activation of cortical areas and is itself influenced by input from the reticular activating system. The consciousness system also influences cortical activity by facilitating or inhibiting sensory information as it is relayed through the thalamus. The cerebral cortex is constantly bombarded by sensory input relayed by the specific thalamic nuclei. Only that sensory input coupled with input from the diffuse projection system identifying it as significant is perceived.

Sleep States

Sleep is also controlled by the consciousness system. Sleep is defined as a cyclic, temporary, and physiological loss of consciousness that is readily, promptly, and completely reversed by appropriate stimuli with no apparent deleterious side effects. Sleep is a behavioral state actively produced and maintained by the consciousness system. It is modulated by exciting the areas of the brain associated with sleep and actively inhibiting the reticular activating system responsible for maintaining wakefulness.

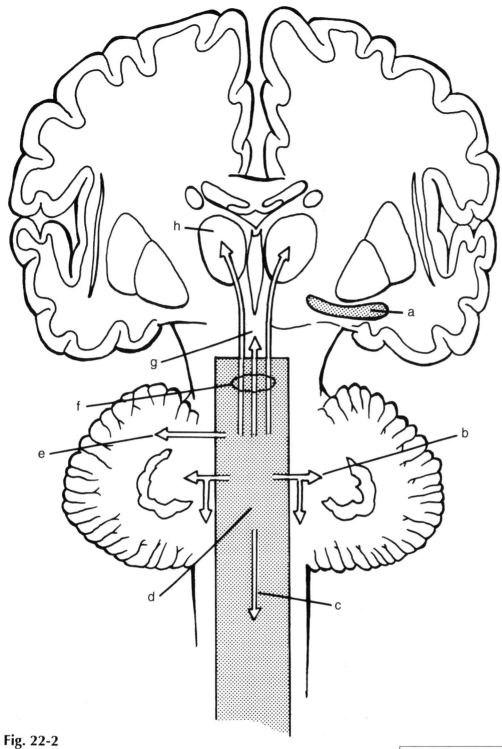

Fig. 22-2

a	Basal forebrain
b	To brain stem nuclei
c	Reticulospinal fibers
d	Brain stem reticular formation
e	To cerebellum
f	Ascending projection fibers
g	Hypothalamus
h	Thalamus

Normal sleep is composed of a recurring pattern of identifiable stages. The primary method for monitoring the stages of sleep is the electroencephalogram (EEG). On the basis of changes in EEG activity, sleep can be subdivided into two distinct patterns, slow-wave sleep (also referred to as non-REM) and rapid eye movement (REM) sleep. Sleep begins with slow-wave sleep, which consists of four stages of progressively deeper sleep. As seen by EEG recordings, the first 30 to 45 minutes are spent progressing through all four stages of slow-wave sleep (Fig. 22-5). EEG patterns show progressively slower-frequency and larger-amplitude activity corresponding to successively deeper states of sleep. During the second 30 to 45 minutes, sleep progresses through the same four steps in reverse order. During slow-wave sleep, no rapid eye movement occurs, muscles are relaxed, and parasympathetic activity predominates. Heart rate, blood pressure, and body temperature decline, and gastrointestinal motility increases. During slow-wave sleep, the deeper the sleep stage the harder it is to awaken the sleeper.

Slow-wave sleep is followed by REM sleep, which is characterized by rapid, conjugate eye movements; fluctuations of heart rate, body temperature, respiration, and blood pressure; penile erection; and involuntary muscle twitching. Dreams occur during REM sleep. An EEG recording at this time reveals rapid, low-amplitude, arrhythmic, and desynchronous cortical activity, indicating that the brain is awake and alert while the body is asleep. Oxygen consumption by the brain is greater during REM sleep than at any other time.

A typical night's sleep pattern involves progressing through alternating cycles of slow-wave and REM stages with REM stages occurring at regular intervals four to six times each night. Throughout the night, the intervals between successive REM periods decrease and the length of each REM period increases. In all, REM sleep occupies approximately 20 to 25 percent of the sleep in young adults. Stage 2 slow-wave sleep occupies approximately 50 percent of the total sleep time, with stages 3 and 4 slow-wave sleep occupying approximately 15 percent.

Slow-wave sleep is mediated by a widespread system that includes multiple groups of neurons (raphe nuclei, nucleus of the solitary tract, reticular nucleus of the thalamus, basal forebrain, anterior hypothalamus, and dorsal medullary reticular formation) that become more active while other neurons in the reticular formation are deactivated. Sleep is also facilitated by serotonergic neurons that decrease sensory input and inhibit motor output from the cortex.

Rapid eye movement sleep is mediated primarily by neurons located ventral and lateral to the locus ceruleus. The midbrain reticular formation and the brain stem tegmentum are also involved. Neurons around the locus ceruleus discharge faster during REM sleep and are called "REM-on cells." The norepinephrine cells of the locus ceruleus and the serotonergic cells in the dorsal raphe nuclei become inactive during REM sleep, and are called the "REM-off cells."

Wake-Sleep States

While it is clear that multiple structures and neuro-humoral agents interact to regulate the cyclic alterations between the wake and sleep states, the precise control mechanisms are not currently understood.

Levels of consciousness correspond to levels of neuronal activity in the cerebral cortex. In the awake, adaptive state, cerebral electrical activity is fast, arrhythmic, desynchronized, and receptive to sensory input. This level of activation reflects the constantly changing input coming from the diffuse thalamocortical projection fibers and medial forebrain bundle as well as thalamocortical input from the sensory systems (including special senses). This excited state is maintained by the activity of cholinergic neurons in the reticular formation and basal forebrain. Norepinephrine neurons of the locus ceruleus increase the activity of cortical and brain stem structures in response to novel stimuli. Histamine neurons in the posterior hypothalamus also enhance the state of wakefulness.

During slow-wave sleep, the wake mechanisms are inhibited and there is decreased responsiveness to external stimuli. The system that regulates slow-wave sleep (raphe nuclei, nucleus of the solitary tract, reticular nucleus of the thalamus, basal forebrain, and anterior hypothalamus) increases activity while other neurons in the reticular formation shut down. Sleep is also facilitated by serotonergic neurons that decrease sensory input and inhibit motor output from the cortex.

Sleep and wakefulness are circadian patterns that occur on approximately a 24-hour cycle. Many other biological functions, including body temperature and hormonal secretion, follow similar patterns. Circadian patterns are set by the "biological clock" located in the suprachiasmatic nucleus of the hypothalamus.

Clinical Aspects

Disorders of Consciousness

Pathological changes in consciousness are produced by major damage to the reticular activating system or cerebral hemispheres bilaterally. Loss of consciousness may be transient or prolonged. If damage occurs in the medulla, the wake and sleep states remain and arousal occurs to appropriate stimulation. If damage occurs above the medullary and pontine sleep centers, there are persistent EEG patterns of wakefulness. If damage occurs at the midbrain, there is a persistent sleep state in which stimulation will not produce arousal. Unilateral lesion of the cerebral hemisphere does not result in loss of consciousness as long as the projections of the consciousness system to at least one cerebral hemisphere are intact.

States of altered consciousness range from normal sleep to brain death. Brain death is the result of irreversible damage that produces unresponsiveness,

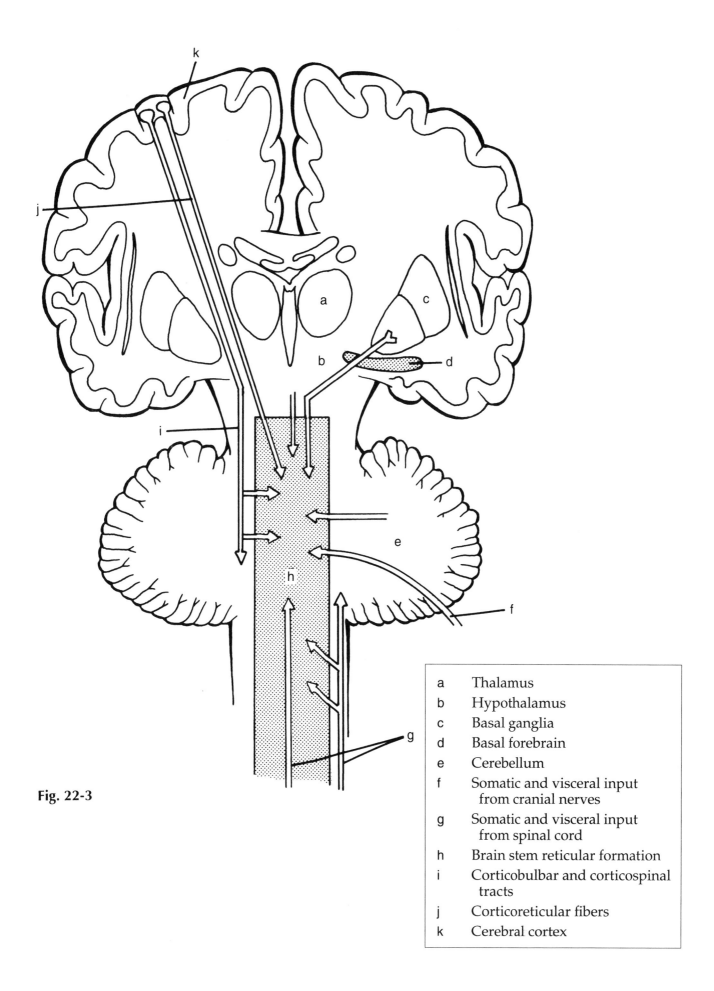

Fig. 22-3

a	Thalamus
b	Hypothalamus
c	Basal ganglia
d	Basal forebrain
e	Cerebellum
f	Somatic and visceral input from cranial nerves
g	Somatic and visceral input from spinal cord
h	Brain stem reticular formation
i	Corticobulbar and corticospinal tracts
j	Corticoreticular fibers
k	Cerebral cortex

with no spontaneous movement or response to external stimuli, absence of all brain stem reflexes including respiration, absence of cerebral blood flow, and absence of cerebral electrical activity (flat EEG). In the presence of brain death, the heart may continue to beat. Coma (a state of extended unconsciousness in which the patient is unarousable, has little or no spontaneous movement, is nonresponsive to stimuli including pain, and has depressed or absent reflexes) is the most severe type of unconsciousness from which people can recover and results from a lesion of the reticular formation and its projection system or the cerebral hemispheres bilaterally. Stupor, obtundation (dulling of the senses), somnolence, and delirium are less severe states of altered consciousness from which individuals may be temporarily aroused. While aroused, responses are appropriate and adaptive. When the stimulation ends, altered consciousness returns. On the way to recovery, patients may pass through several of these stages.

Concussion, seizure, syncope (fainting), and metabolic encephalopathy may all cause unconsciousness, but most tend to produce no permanent neuronal damage. Severe concussions may produce diffuse axonal injury as seen in some closed head injuries. Toxic or anoxic metabolic encephalopathy, on the other hand, may produce severe and irreversible brain damage with severe functional deficiencies.

Sleep Disorders

Lesions of the raphe nuclei, or pharmacological agents that block serotonin synthesis, cause a reduction of slow-wave sleep and result in insomnia. Lesions of the locus ceruleus or disruption of norepinephrine synthesis allow a person to fall asleep and enter slow-wave sleep, but shorten the duration of the REM sleep period.

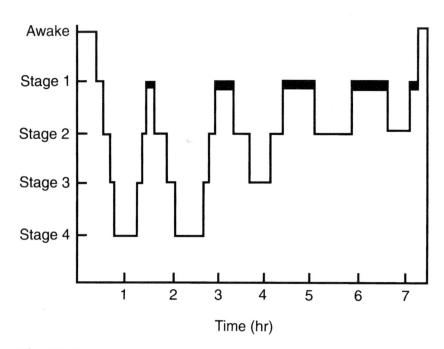

Fig. 22-5

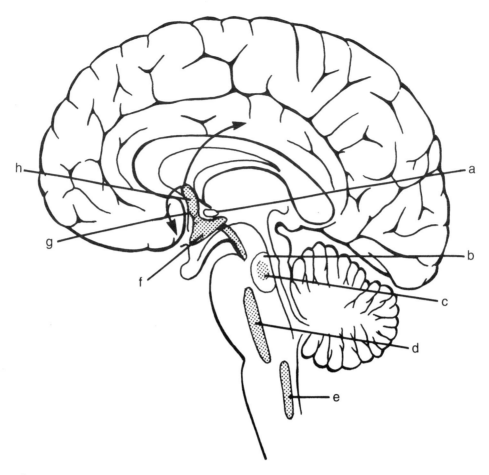

Fig. 22-4

a	Anterior hypothalamic nucleus
b	Dorsolateral pons
c	Locus ceruleus
d	Raphe nuclei
e	Nucleus solitarius
f	Nucleus basalis
g	Medial forebrain bundle
h	Septal nucleus

Index